MEASURING HEALTH FROM THE INSIDE

Nutrition, Metabolism & Body Composition

BY CAROLYN HODGES CHAFFEE, MS, RDN, CEDRD
& ANNIKA KAHM, MS

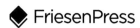

FriesenPress

Suite 300 - 990 Fort St
Victoria, BC, Canada, V8V 3K2
www.friesenpress.com

ISBN
978-1-4602-5859-0 (Paperback)
978-1-4602-5860-6 (eBook)

1. Psychology, Psychopathology, Eating Disorders

Distributed to the trade by The Ingram Book Company

DEDICATION

To my parents who provided me with invaluable guidance
and support and to my children who have always believed in me.
Carolyn

To my mother who always supported and believed in me,
and for my children and grandchildren who inspire me.
Annika

Finally, we dedicate this book to you, to all our patients,
with love and appreciation.
Thanks for trusting us and for allowing us to be part of your life.
Carolyn & Annika

"As someone who has both worked professionally in the eating disorders field and benefited immensely from the treatment modalities described in Carolyn and Annika's book, I am excited and grateful to have this clearly written tool available to clinicians treating eating disorders and families and individuals personally affected by them. I cannot understate the life changing benefits I have directly experienced as a result of Metabolic Testing and Body Composition Analysis being added to my eating disorder treatment. So many unanswered questions about my body were answered, enabling me to trust my treatment team and take solid steps to heal my body from years of deprivation. Those struggling from eating disorders deserve to have access to the type of information outlined in this book, and the standard of care available through the addition of the MT and BCA tests to treatment protocol should be a goal for every clinician."

Joslyn P. Smith
Eating Disorder and Health At Every Size^R Advocate

*""You can't do anything different, until you see it differently." It was from that lens that changed how I responded to my daughters eating disorders. My family was no longer navigating this disease in the dark. We could see beyond the shame, stigma and the scale. **Measuring Health From The Inside** is a profound book that will forever change how we see and treat this devastating disease. This book reveals the truth about our bodies' needs and invites us to be part of the healing and recovery process. **Measuring Health From The Inside** is for... everyBODY."*

Mary Ellen Clausen
Parent and Founder of Ophelia's Place

"Incorporating up-to-date research on the intricacies of the full range of eating disorders, Hodges-Chaffee' and Kahm's sophististicated but accessible book provides patients and families with a respectfully collaborative approach to understanding and treating these challenging illnesses."

Douglas W. Bunnell, Ph.D., FEAD, CEDS
Chief Clinical Development and Education Officer Monte Nido & Affiliated

"*Measuring Health From The Inside* is a must-read for both individuals and families suffering from eating disorders, as well as the health care professionals treating them. Carolyn Hodges - Chaffee and Annika Kahm present a ground breaking approach to moving beyond the standard weights and labs, and look inside the body for a true measure of malnutrition and the impact of the eating disorder on the body. This is an excellent guide to help individuals understand the impact of malnutrition on the recovery process and seek out an appropriate treatment team."

Christy Duffy, Ph.D.
HSPP Director, Under the Umbrella

"*Measuring Health From The Inside* is an innovative approach to understanding the science behind food choices, eating behaviors and how these impact the body in terms of health, energy, weight management and more. Beyond BMI, body fat percentages and weight, the authors introduce a much needed expansion and refinement of measurement techniques to the nutrition arm of eating disorder treatment. They do this using easily understandable language and clear cut data that the general population as a whole will find incredibly useful and applicable."

Sonya Rencevicz, LCSW

"In *Measuring Health from the Inside* Carolyn Hodges Chaffee and Annika Kahm have clearly outlined their clinical nutrition practice of performing metabolic testing and body composition analysis with eating disorder patients. Their approach bridges the gap between science and patient education by providing these challenging patients with actual data about their specific bodies. By giving patients these data, they can begin to understand the specific effects that restriction, purging and binge eating each have on the body. I have personally sent refractory patients to Annika for these exact reasons. It is my hope that more nutritionists will use these methods in the future."

Rachel S-D Fortune, MD, FAAP
Medical Director, Newport Academy

"*Measuring Health from The Inside* is a brilliant and necessary addition to the Clinician's tool box for treating Eating Disorders. The authors present a straightforward yet comprehensive methodology for enrolling the patient in their own recovery. Through their case studies we enter these patient's lives and feel the agony of an eating disorder. The authors show that with compassion and data, patients can be motivated to partner in their own recovery. Written with conviction and years of experience, *Measuring Health from The Inside* shows when an eating disorder is present, how diagnoses are made and how treatment should be delivered in today's data rich environment. This instructive book reminds us that the stories of our eating disordered patients always matter and are never without the possibility of a happy end."

Dr Joanna Bronfman, LCSW, Psy.D.
Founder and Clinical Director of Backcountry Wellness, LLC

"*This remarkable book represents the distillation of literally decades of experience of two gifted senior clinicians addressing the crucial nutritional aspects of eating disorders. It is characterized by a structured, clear, concise, and accessible style and illustrated by appropriately focused clinical anecdotes. The work is largely (but not exclusively) organized around the use of two diagnostic tests - Metabolic Testing and Body Composition Analysis . Aside from their intrinsic value in informing and guiding the course of treatment, the authors have also found these tests particularly valuable for engaging patients as collaborators in the treatment, helping them to understand the rationale for each aspect of treatment strategy, and making it possible for them to see concrete evidence of even early progress as the treatment unfolds. The result is a coherent and carefully designed approach to understanding and constructively addressing the nutritional treatment eating disorders. Whether approached as a comprehensive text or as a reference work, the reader will be consistently rewarded with useful observations and ingenious solutions to common clinical dilemmas.*"

David Greenfeld M.D.
Clinical Professor of Psychiatry, Yale University School of Medicine

*"**Measuring Health From The Inside** is spot on as a comprehensive introduction to eating disorders for both families as well as professional caregivers. Where it separates and distinguishes itself from other books of its nature is its emphasis on using metabolic testing and body composition analysis as a measure to determine an individual's appropriate nutritional health. In the world of eating disorders this is traditionally determined by the number on the scale which leads to much subjectivity from the patient on what that appropriate number should be. Metabolic testing and body composition analysis takes the number on the scale out of the equation and uses concrete measures to help the individual understand how their eating behaviors are directly affecting their bodies in both a positive and negative way."*

John Samanich MD., MS.

Director of Child and Adolescent Psychiatry, Greenwich Child & Adolescent Psychiatry, LLC

"As a Psychologist with a background in nursing this book is ground breaking in its explanation of essential nutritional tools, and the application of physiology in treating ED illnesses. I would recommend it to all disciplines treating Eating Disorders. I would also recommend this insightful book to clients in recovery, and their families. This is crucial scientific information that is easily understandable and essential in recovery. My experience is that the methods of the writers decrease anxiety in an illness that is fear and distortion based"

Cindy James, R.N., Ph.D.

over 30 years in field of ED

CONTENTS

Dedication..i

Acknowledgements ix

Preface xi

Foreword
by Diane Mickley, MD xiii

Introduction
Measuring Health from the Inside... xv

Chapter 1 Malnutrition..1
Bringing Malnutrition into the Conversation.....................................1
Identifying Malnutrition..4
The Importance of Serotonin...8
The Usefulness of Metabolic
Testing and Body Composition Analysis 9

Chapter 2 The Eating Disorder Voice.. 11
The Effects of a Starving Brain 11
How Obsessive-Compulsive Thoughts Evolve into the Eating Disorder Voice12
Biochemical Changes in the Brain when the Body Is Underfed......................13
Increased Obsessive-Compulsive Thoughts 15
Psychotropic Medication 15
Why Obsessive-Compulsive Thoughts Increase When Normal Eating
Resumes...16

Chapter 3 Metabolic Testing and Body Composition Analysis....................19
Metabolism...20
Measuring Metabolic Rate..22
Metabolic Testing: Analyzing the Results 23
Body Composition Analysis...26
Taking the Guesswork out of Treatment..28

Chapter 4 Anorexia Nervosa..31
Dangerous Mindset, Dangerous Habits 31
The Image in the Mirror...32
Identifying Anorexia Nervosa..33

Denial is Part of the Disease 36
Current Trends in Anorexia Nervosa 36
Usefulness of Metabolic Testing and Body Composition Analysis 39

Chapter 5 Bulimia Nervosa **43**
Exposing the Secrets of Bulimia Nervosa 44
The Fallout from Purging 44
Prescreening, Diagnosing, and Treating Bulimia Nervosa 45
Warning Signs of Bulimia Nervosa 46
Beyond the Warning Signs 46
The Usefulness of Metabolic Testing and Body Composition Analysis 50

Chapter 6 Binge Eating Disorder **53**
I Just Can't Stop Myself 53
Why Does Someone Binge? 54
Identifying Binge Eating Disorder 55
Warning Signs of Binge Eating Disorder 56
Beyond the Warning Signs 56
The Usefulness of Metabolic Testing and Body Composition Analysis 57
Treatment Protocols for BED 59

Chapter 7 Compulsive Exercise **62**
When Endorphins Meet the Eating Disorder Voice 62
Giving Compulsive Exercise the Attention it Deserves 63
Identifying Compulsive Exercise 63
The Terminology 64
Brain Changes 65
Cortisol: The Feared Hormone 67
The Role of the Eating Disorder Voice 67
Warning Signs of Compulsive Exercise 68
Beyond the Warning Signs 68
Relative Energy Deficit in Sports (RED-S) 70
The Usefulness of Metabolic Testing and Body Composition Analysis 71

Chapter 8 Other Specified Feeding and Eating Disorders (OSFED) **75**
OSFED Sub-Types 76
OSFED Disorders 77
Challenges with Treating OSFED Patients 79
The Usefulness of Metabolic Testing and Body Composition Analysis 81

Chapter 9

Healthy Eating **86**
Nutrition: The Cornerstone of Our Practices 86
What the Body Needs to Function 87
A Balanced Food Plan 87

The Usefulness of Metabolic Testing and Body Composition Analysis..........90
The Importance of Breakfast and Front-Loading Calories............................92
The Need to Consume More Calories...93
Changing Energy Levels..93
Signs the Body Is Repairing Itself...94

Chapter 10 Treatment Protocols and Higher Levels of Care......................**98**
Treatment Team: Taking a Multidisciplinary Approach....................................98
Recommendations for Those Seeking Treatment..99
Outpatient Treatment Protocol..99
When a Higher Level of Care is Necessary...101
Selecting a Treatment Program...103

Chapter 11 Recovery: Why It's Not a Linear Process..............................**107**
Recovery is a Process...107
Early Recovery Stage...108
Ongoing Recovery..111
Fully Recovered..113
Resiliency...116

Chapter 12 Final Thoughts: From Small Steps to Milestones.....................**119**
Sustained Recovery: From Our Perspective...119
You Can't Do Anything Different, Until You See it Differently.......................120

Notes..**125**

Index..**134**

ACKNOWLEDGEMENTS

We would like to thank the following people who have helped us make this book a reality:

Carl Bennet for his remarkable generosity sponsoring the publishing of the book.

Dr. Ruben Cuadrado who was Carolyn's mentor for several years. He co-founded the Nutrition Clinic and was instrumental in recognizing the need for Metabolic Testing and Body Composition Analysis to provide a thorough and accurate nutritional assessment of patients.

Dr. Marc Immerman, Medical Director of the Nutrition Clinic. His ongoing support has allowed us to grow into a program that treats several hundred patients annually.

Our friends Gunilla and Len Vickers who whole-heartedly supported the idea to write a book and who helped us refine its ideas. Gunilla gave so much of her time and wisdom, helped organizing ideas as well as providing constant support.

Carolyn's sister Sue, who provided guidance and professional expertise as well as much time and effort to help recognize the initial shortcomings, organize and edit the book.

Annika's son Nick, who gave continuous and honest critique and who guided us to find the right editor.

Diane Mickley, MD, who is recognizing the importance of Body Composition Analysis and Metabolic Testing. Not only did she willingly write the foreword, but she also added valuable input regarding the content of the book.

Sheila Buff who assisted with the editing and organization of the book.

Our colleagues who provided invaluable guidance and support throughout the process.

FriesenPress who not only guided us, but made sure our work finally became a book.

We are also greatly indebted to the many patients and their families whose stories and struggles have both taught and inspired us and we want to thank them all for putting their faith and hope in our abilities.

And last, but not the least, we thank those patients who have generously shared their stories and who trusted us in their journey towards recovery.

PREFACE

We are two nutritionists who have over 70 years of combined experience treating a broad range of eating disorders.

We met at a conference several years ago, where Carolyn presented an innovative way of doing nutritional assessments. Using two medical devices, Carolyn was able to measure what was going on inside her patients' bodies. She was no longer limited to the information that nutritionists and medical doctors routinely use to assess health. Because Carolyn could assess her patient's nutritional health with far greater accuracy, she could offer far more effective, customized treatments. This opened Annika's eyes and she transformed her practice accordingly. Since then, we have often collaborated. Annika has seen a tremendous improvement in the quality of care she is now able to offer.

But we have been disappointed that these useful assessment tools and practices remain virtually unknown among the general public, doctors, nutritionists, and other specialists. The purpose of this book is to disseminate this knowledge to improve the current treatment of eating disorders. We offer this book as a starting point in the hope that these treatment tools and practices will become more widely known and used, that the book will spur further research, and that it may answer questions for practitioners and patients who wish to offer or obtain better treatment.

By writing this book, we hope clinicians, patients, and families will realize the types of diagnostic testing that are available to measure an individual's nutritional health when an eating disorder is suspected. Yes, it is easy to recognize when someone has low body weight and is in need of nutritional support, but what about someone who is normal weight, above-normal weight, or obese, especially when all blood work is within a normal range? How can you tell if an individual is malnourished? Metabolic Testing and Body Composition Analysis are two diagnostic tests that help measure health from inside the body. Both of our practices rely on these two types of tests to ensure we have the best data possible when diagnosing and treating our patients.

The testing provides an assessment of health that patients have not seen before. During the follow-up visits, we are able to evaluate the severity of the eating disorder and present them with clear-cut data. The test results not only show them tangible information they can understand, but it also motivates our patients to make the recommended changes. Throughout the treatment, these are invaluable tools that help guide us in correcting the body's nutritional status. Too often, patients hear the message that they must be better because they are not at a low body weight and "don't look sick." Metabolic Testing and Body Composition Analysis help assess health from the inside and can actually assist us in determining when the body is repaired.

Our combined practices have treated over 8,000 patients with this methodology. It has allowed us to be much more aggressive in our approach, shortens the length of treatment time, allows us to identify malnutrition much sooner, and has improved treatment outcomes. Initially, we used this type of testing to assess eating disorder and disordered eating patients, but we have now expanded our practices to include all types of individuals seeking nutritional counseling for a variety of problems, including fatigue, autoimmune diseases, sports performance, anxiety, depression, sensory issues that interfere with eating, cancer, weight loss, and bariatric patients. We truly believe Metabolic Testing and Body Composition Analysis should be part of an individual's annual health physical. Metabolic Testing and Body Composition Analysis have radically improved our ability to successfully treat our patients. We cannot imagine going back to the time when the scale was our primary method of assessing health.

FOREWORD
by Diane Mickley, MD

Eating disorders are notoriously difficult illnesses—a fact known too well by patients, families, and the clinicians who treat them. Anorexia Nervosa and Bulimia Nervosa can be insidious and invisible. They often are accompanied by a false sense of physical wellbeing. Physical exams and blood tests are often fairly normal. Yet eating disorders can be chronic or even deadly. The bright note in this is that eating disorders are potentially curable, but this is most likely to occur with specialized and knowledgeable care, early in the illness and through to complete recovery. Yet many patients don't get the best treatments available, and even those who do can have a long and hard struggle.

Measuring Health from the Inside shines a light on a valuable addition to the treatment of eating disorders: Metabolic Testing and Body Composition Analysis. These are noninvasive assessments with immediate results. The results show patients numerically and graphically if they have slowed their metabolism and if they are burning off muscle for lack of fuel. The testing provides objective data on how many calories the patient needs, as well as what is an accurate ideal weight. Eating disorders often play tricks with the thinking of the very bright people who are especially vulnerable to them. Nutritional assessment avoids much of the debate about what is the real health status of the patient and what he/she needs dietarily to get well.

Annika Kahm and Carolyn Chaffee bring decades of expertise in the care of patients with classic Anorexia Nervosa, Bulimia Nervosa, Binge Eating Disorder, and the many related atypical and subsyndromal variants (OSFED, or Other Specified Eating and Feeding Disorders). Their clinical wisdom, understanding of the experience of sufferers and those who love them, and understanding of these illnesses and the recovery process infuse these pages. Their perspective, techniques, and strategies will be an asset to everyone who seeks to eradicate eating disorders—in themselves or their patients.

Measuring Health from the Inside highlights the invaluable benefits of Metabolic Testing and Body Composition, and their value in skilled hands to promote understanding of the physiologic effects of eating disorders and the nutritional requirements for recovery. Kudos to the authors for the gift of this information.

Diane Mickley, MD, FACP, FAED
Director, Wilkins Center for Eating Disorders
Assistant Clinical Professor, Department of Psychiatry,
Yale University School of Medicine

INTRODUCTION

Measuring Health from the Inside

Eating disorders are increasing at an alarming rate. The death rate for Anorexia Nervosa in the U.S. is 12 times higher than all other leading causes of death combined for the 15 to 24 age group.[1] Many dynamics contribute to this exponential change, including environmental factors and societal pressures. Additionally, research has shown genetics can often be a major contributor. However, the present treatment modalities for eating disorders are severely lacking and the field remains understudied.

Our goal in writing this book is to illustrate the innovative way we diagnose and treat patients with eating disorders. Simultaneously, we want to provide the reader with a better understanding of the important role malnutrition plays in the manifestation of this disease. Through this discussion, we strongly feel we can add to the body of literature that already exists on eating disorders—specifically on treatment modalities. Overall, we hope to advocate that health should be measured from the inside and urge practitioners to use more than the individual's body weight and blood work when assessing and treating this disease.

We are not researchers. We are clinicians with over 70 years of combined experience in treating and supervising the treatment of more than 8,000 patients who struggle with eating disorders. This book highlights case studies, patient testimonials, and anecdotal observations. It also outlines our protocol when diagnosing and treating this population. Hopefully, the result will offer a better understanding of the treatment protocols we have used, protocols that have not only had positive and extremely effective outcomes but also have ultimately resulted in thousands of success stories.

The first two chapters of this book discuss our approach in understanding how an eating disorder develops and how malnutrition and the "eating disorder voice" go hand in hand in becoming major contributors to the onset of this disease. We also discuss how biochemical changes occur in the body when it is underfed. In our view, the need to carefully screen for malnutrition, diagnose it properly, and then effectively treat it is essential when treating this population. This provides the basic knowledge needed to understand why it is necessary to measure health from the inside.

The nuts and bolts of our approach to actually measure health from the inside is discussed in chapter three as we describe our use of Metabolic Testing (indirect calorimetry) and Body Composition Analysis. These two critical tests are a standard part of our practice. For over 20 years, we have been using them to test each and every patient who comes to us for treatment to prescreen for malnutrition. Including this in our prescreening protocol has led to our successful outcomes and we strongly urge all clinicians to begin incorporating this into their practice. Unfortunately, this treatment modality seems to be rarely used. By writing this book, we hope to change that. Furthermore, we argue this should be part of any individual's nutritional assessment, and should be included in an annual health physical. If a health practitioner is not offering these two tests, we hope to encourage individuals who are seeking treatment to find one who does.

As nutritionists, we have knowledge and understanding about what happens to the body when it is malnourished and how malnutrition can develop into an eating disorder. Unfortunately, nutrition—or in this case, malnutrition—is an area that has not been adequately explored. We often hear of malnutrition in underdeveloped countries, but what about the United States? Malnutrition does not discriminate; it can and does affect many more individuals than is realized. It is not difficult to identify an individual who has extremely low body weight and diagnose him or her with malnutrition, but what about normal or above-normal body weights? Malnutrition can affect anyone, anytime, and in any place.

As we discuss in chapter one, malnutrition is often missed as being a key factor when analyzing and researching eating disorders. We contend this is the reason many clinicians overlook the need to test for malnutrition, leaving the patient misdiagnosed (sometimes for several years). This does not mean that everyone who is malnourished has an eating disorder, but it does mean that they will eventually suffer medical consequences as a result of being malnourished.

Metabolic Testing and Body Composition Analysis have been available for years, the former since the late 1700s and the latter since the mid-1980s. What these tests allow us to do is individualize treatment, because no two patients are the same. Why is it some individuals become malnourished very quickly and show signs of it, while other individuals can under-eat for years and still maintain a normal or above-normal body weight? These are areas that need to be researched. Crow and colleagues found that the mortality rate is actually higher in the "Eating Disorder, Not Otherwise Specified" group than in Anorexia Nervosa or Bulimia Nervosa groups.[2] Why is it that these groups of patients receive the least amount of care? Just because they "don't look sick" doesn't mean that they aren't. Metabolic Testing and Body Composition Analysis take the guesswork out of identifying who is and who is not malnourished.

As described in chapter three, the data obtained through these tests helps us determine how aggressive our care needs to be. We are able to identify malnourished individuals much sooner. This also helps when trying to motivate patients to make the changes we are prescribing. When they are unable to follow the treatment recommendations prescribed, we see this as an indication that they may need a higher level of care.

As seen in the patient testimonials included throughout the book, the feedback we receive is overwhelming positive. Patients tell us, **"This data is so helpful, I always thought what I was doing was healthy," "I never would have believed I wasn't eating enough until I saw these tests,"** and **"I can actually trust the recommendations because I can see how my body has been working."** While these testimonials might seem anecdotal, we see them as sound qualitative data on the effectiveness of incorporating Metabolic Testing and Body Composition Analysis into our treatment protocol.

Measurement of recovery is often focused on the weight of the individual, but it cannot be understated that *body weight tells us very little*. An individual may have returned to their normal or ideal body weight but can still be malnourished. Incorporating these tests help clinicians avoid the pitfall of arguing with the patient about their target or ideal body weight. When the tests results show that the body is no longer malnourished, then, and only then, can it be said that an appropriate weight has been reached.

Improving nutritional status can and will shorten the length of treatment time. Individuals who are receiving weekly therapy, but who are still binging and purging or restricting, will benefit more from therapy when they are nutritionally supported. We see many individuals who are weight-restored, but still malnourished. We have also seen patients who have been told that they have not responded to medication trials, but were not nutritionally assessed. Maybe the poor response to the medication was because the individual was malnourished. We know our brain functions much better when it is fed. We have seen obsessive thoughts significantly decrease in the individual who is nutritionally supported, but remain very strong in those that are malnourished.

The mid-section of this book (chapters four through eight) discuss the different types of eating disorders. They contain question-and-answer sections that provide a more in-depth understanding of each individual disorder. We include the warning signs and a subsection on "beyond the warning signs" that covers the physiological and psychological complications associated with each of the different eating disorders.

The last third of this book focuses on our treatment plan, and includes a discussion on nutrition and healthy eating and how we apply this knowledge when treating our patients through each stage of their treatment—from our initial assessment through to full recovery. Chapter 10 provides a synopsis of our recommendations for a treatment protocol, including the need to put together a multidisciplinary treatment team to work with patients. In this same chapter we move the discussion into the options for higher levels of care when the patient is not responding to an outpatient treatment program.

This section also provides an in-depth review of what recovery entails and how it is not a linear process. We think this section is particularly important for family members and friends of the patient to read because having them understand that recovery is not a linear process helps them not to judge or be critical when there are slip-ups or relapses. As we point out in this chapter, recovery is a very fluid process; some days are good and others are more of a struggle. One of our goals in writing this chapter was to provide a better understanding of the different dynamics, both physiological and psychological, that can either make recovery smooth or make it a challenge.

And finally, chapter 12 highlights the sense of accomplishment and relief many of our patients feel once they are fully recovered. The testimonials in this chapter give a voice to some of those patients who have a sense of renewal in their lives. We've also included some milestone markers or memorable moments for us as clinicians. This is a very rewarding patient population to work with and seeing the changes they are able to achieve keeps us determined to provide state-of-the-art care for better treatment outcomes.

Once again, we want to emphasize nutritional support should be a cornerstone of treatment, not an adjunct. Nutritional status is critical at every stage of working with patients, from developing their individualized treatment plan to analyzing when the body has completely recovered. It is our hope that by urging practitioners to measure health from the inside, our work can have an impact on improving current trends in treatment modalities, something that is seriously needed in this field.

CHAPTER 1

Malnutrition

We often hear about malnutrition when discussing nutrition in underdeveloped countries, but what about the United States? For the most part, there is research in the United States on the effects of poverty and the high incidences of food insecurity that can result in malnutrition; but what about when there is an abundance of food? In addition, what about circumstances where individuals have seemingly healthy eating behaviors, but still become malnourished and develop an eating disorder? Because there is often an overlap between malnutrition and eating disorders, it is important to broaden the discussion to explore this nexus, and to have a better understanding of what malnutrition does to the body.

BRINGING MALNUTRITION INTO THE CONVERSATION

In our practices, we initially nutritionally assess a patient and determine if they are in a hypometabolic (a slowed metabolism) and/or catabolic state (using their own protein stores) since both of these can indicate malnutrition. This is not normal protocol for most practitioners. As nutritionists, we know how much the body is affected by starvation or an inadequate food intake and that full recovery greatly depends on malnutrition being quickly identified and addressed. Positive treatment outcomes depend on how early the intervention is and how quickly the body can be restored. If the eating disorder is successfully treated, the body can be healed and return to normal.

Therefore, the discussion needs to be broadened whenever eating disorders are the topic and should definitely encompass malnutrition. Not only do researchers and practitioners need to have a complete understanding of hypometabolic and catabolic states, but they should also be knowledgeable about the psychological and physiological effects malnutrition has on the body, especially when this is coupled with an eating disorder. In addition, we also contend the conversation needs to include discussions of how and when perceived healthy eating behaviors develop into malnutrition and how this leads to an eating disorder.

Minnesota Starvation Experiment

To better understand the physiological and psychological effects of severe and prolonged starvation, Ancel Keys carried out a starvation study during World War II with 36 conscientious male objectors who were healthy volunteers. The entire study lasted one year and included three months of an initial control period, six months of semi-starvation, and three months of re-feeding. Extensive testing was done at each stage and during the following year. The semi-starvation diet, averaging 1,570 kcal, was less than half the amount eaten during the control period (3,200 kcal). This caused a 25 percent reduction in body weight, decreased metabolic rate, decreased heart rate, slowed respiration (breathing), dizziness, hair loss, and lowered body temperature. Mentally, the subjects experienced severe emotional distress, depression, mood-swings and difficulty in thinking and comprehension. They became preoccupied with food, collecting recipes and preplanning meals. Although 1,500 calories may not sound like starvation, it nevertheless resulted in devastating effects to the body and brain.

The physical effects of the induced semi-starvation closely resemble the conditions experienced by people with a wide range of eating disorders. As a result of the study, researchers have postulated that many of the psychological effects of eating disorders may result from undernutrition, and recovery depends on re-feeding as well as psychological treatment.[1]

The Nexus between Malnutrition and Eating Disorders

Which comes first—malnutrition or an eating disorder? It is almost intuitive to suspect individuals would become malnourished when their food intake is severely restricted or the majority of it is purged; but is this the only time there is a connection between malnutrition and an eating disorder? Malnutrition can be brought on by many different ways beyond severely restricting food intake or purging. For example, individuals who exercise and do not adequately fuel their body can become nutritionally depleted. Individuals who restrict there overall intake and eat the majority of their food later in the day may not be low body weight but can become malnourished. The body adapts to being underfed by slowing down to preserve itself and then uses vital stores to take care of its nutritional needs—ultimately resulting in a malnourished body.

So when and how do normal eating behaviors develop into an eating disorder? Usually there is a period of time when one or several irregular eating behaviors are present that can cause physical or psychological changes. This disordered eating can be a result of wanting to lose weight, maintaining a specific weight, or managing emotions, and can lead to an eating disorder. Our experience has shown that disordered eating becomes a problem when the behaviors interfere with being able to eat and maintain health and/or daily functioning.

We often see individuals who think their eating behaviors are leading them to good health when in fact their food behaviors are leading them to malnourishment. The physical consequences of malnutrition in a seemingly healthy body not only leads to nutritional deficiencies but has also resulted in Anorexia Nervosa, Bulimia Nervosa, Binge Eating Disorder, and Other Specified Feeding and Eating Disorders (OSFED).

Typical Food Behaviors of Our Patients
- Limited food choices
- Dieting
- Using over-the-counter or online dieting products

- Fasting or cleansing to lose weight
- Skipping meals
- Eliminating food groups
- Becoming vegan or vegetarian to avoid eating many foods
- High level of exercise while restricting food intake

IDENTIFYING MALNUTRITION

Malnutrition in a normal-weight or above normal-weight individual is very difficult to identify. While vague complaints such as feeling tired or more depressed may be an indicator, we recommend Metabolic Testing with this patient population. This test not only measures what is going on inside the body, but it can also show if the patient's body is using its own reserves to fuel itself. Metabolic Testing can also reveal when a body is in a hypometabolic state or a catabolic state.

Hypometabolic and Catabolic States

A hypometabolic state occurs when the body slows down as a result of inadequate food intake and cannot meet its own nutritional needs. A catabolic state occurs when the body uses its own protein stores to meet its nutritional needs. If the body is in this state just briefly, it adapts and there are no long-term consequences. However, if it is in the starved state for a longer period of time, the adaptation can result in significant protein losses. Non-adapted, protein-calorie malnutrition is dangerous and can compromise muscles of the heart and respiratory system as well as compromise the immune system.[2]

The following case study is an example of how incorporating Metabolic Testing into our treatment protocol allows us to quickly identify when a patient is malnourished, and in a hypometabolic and catabolic state.

C.B.'s Story

C. B. is a 46-year-old female who was training for a marathon. She was frustrated because despite a high level of exercise her weight had increased 15 pounds over the past year. She was hoping that training for the marathon would help her lose weight. C. B. typically ate approximately 1,500 calories a day and was running 6 to 8 miles a day and 12 miles on the weekend. Metabolic Testing showed she was severely hypometabolic, burning only 583 calories per day, with normal being 2200-2400 calories. She was catabolic, with a protein substrate utilization of 48 percent, normal being 15 percent. When shown the results, she was in disbelief. How could she be burning only 583 calories a day when she was running at least 45 to 60 minutes daily? She said, "I can't be malnourished, I'm overweight!" (She was 5'7" and weighed 155 pounds.) Her blood work showed signs of malnutrition, her white blood cell count was low, and she was slightly anemic. There had also been increased hair loss and she felt like she was "losing her mind." She could not remember things that typically came easily to her, and she had not previously had a problem with memory. She attributed this to the normal aging process. She felt increased fatigue because she was exercising more and drank more coffee to keep her energy level up.

Without Metabolic Testing, C. B. would have never believed she was malnourished or that she would have to eat more to feel better. Reluctantly, she increased her calorie intake to 2,500 calories. Within a short period of time, she had more energy and her running times improved. Over the next eight weeks she continued to run, and increased her intake to 3,000 calories a day. Within a few months her memory, focus, and concentration also improved, along with her performance. Her metabolism took approximately three months to totally correct. It takes much longer for a body to correct a malnourished state when an individual continues to exercise. She is now a believer, saying, "I've got to eat enough calories to compensate for my activity level. If I don't, I can do serious damage to my brain and body."

Physiological Changes and Complications

Prescreening individuals for the physiological changes they have been experiencing is also recommended when trying to identify whether or not a patient is malnourished. The body's basic metabolic response to starvation is to conserve body tissues and energy. However, the body will use its own stores to meet its needs if food is not present, including muscle and organ tissue.[3] Also, loss of body fat below a critical mass is a serious issue. The body uses fat during starvation as a protective mechanism to provide glucose substrate for organs that must have glucose to allow life to continue. Death from starvation is due to total fat depletion because there are no more fatty acids available for gluconeogenesis and ketone bodies.[4]

The following problems and complications are also prevalent in malnourished and eating disordered populations:

> *Gastrointestinal complaints.* Common gastrointestinal complaints include feeling full, bloating, constipation, diarrhea, reflux, cramping, and abdominal pain. These are typically caused by the food restriction, binging, purging, and laxative use. Gastroparesis, delayed emptying of the stomach, occurs when there is a weight loss of approximately 10 to 20 pounds.[5]

> *Cardiac complications.* Cardiac complications can include an irregular or abnormally slow heart rate, which can mean the heart muscle is undergoing changes. This can lead to low blood pressure, a slow heart rate (bradycardia, a heart rate of less than 60 beats per minute), and heart failure.[6]

> *Loss of protein matrix tissue.* The loss of protein matrix tissue (density) from bones, which leaves them brittle and susceptible to fracture, is an indicator that osteoporosis is present. Research shows that osteoporosis is present

in almost 40 percent of female patients with Anorexia Nervosa, and osteopenia is present in 92 percent of these women.[7] Although this is a disease that typically affects the elderly, individuals who restrict their intake, have amenorrhea (absence of the menstrual cycle), and low calcium or phosphate intake, may be at a high risk. This puts individuals at a much higher risk for stress fractures and poor healing.

Immune system damage. The body's immune system also becomes compromised when the body is malnourished. Low white blood cell count can occur, increasing the body's vulnerability to infection.

Other physical complaints. Other physical complaints can include impaired wound healing (low calorie and protein intake affects the body's ability to heal), a drop in the body's basal temperature, and disturbed sleep. The skin also shows signs of malnutrition. It can bruise easily, is dry, and growth of fine hair all over the body (lunago) can occur.[8]

Other physiological reasons that can lead to the development of malnutrition may need to be ruled out before an eating disorder can be identified. Medical illnesses may mimic or present as an eating disorder. Gastrointestinal illnesses such as celiac disease, ulcerative colitis, chronic parasites, and malabsorption need to be ruled out. Endocrine disorders including diabetes mellitus, Addison's disease, hyperthyroidism, hypopituitarism, and cancers can mimic an eating disorder. It is also important to understand that there is an increased risk of developing an eating disorder with diabetes mellitus, attention deficit disorder, celiac disease, gastric bypass, and other illnesses that require the restriction or regulation of food intake.[9]

Neurological and Psychological Changes and Complications

Prescreening for neurological and psychological changes is also necessary since impaired brain function can alter mood, judgment, behavior, cognition, personality, and autonomic nervous system control in malnourished and eating disordered populations.[10] It is important to fully understand that the worse the malnutrition is, the more harmful it will be to the brain. And subsequently, the more affected the brain is, the more the mind will be affected, making the eating disorder worse as well.

Brain functional magnetic resonance imaging (fMRI) scans have shown changes in gray and white matter of the brain caused by malnutrition, suggesting a degree of cerebral atrophy. The changes in white matter have been shown to reverse with weight restoration, whereas gray matter volume deficits and blood flow disturbances often persist.. Neurological changes that occur as a result of malnutrition also include apathy and poor concentration.[11]

Other neurological and psychological complications associated with malnourishment in eating disordered patients include:

> *Cognitive problems.* Cognitive problems caused by malnutrition can include a lack of attention span, concentration, memory, and visuospatial ability. Individuals with Anorexia Nervosa and Bulimia Nervosa also struggle with a distorted or delusional perception of the body.[12]

> *Compulsive thoughts.* As food intake decreases, incessant, compulsive thoughts about what to eat and not eat increase. Medication for the treatment of the eating disorder and co-occurring illnesses will not be as effective until the body is nourished.[13] The malnutrition needs to be treated in order to determine what other psychiatric and physical problems need to be addressed.

THE IMPORTANCE OF SEROTONIN

Individuals begin to restrict their intake of food for many reasons. The most common ones we hear in our practices are, **"I just wanted to eat healthier,"** or **"I just wanted to lose a few pounds."** Regardless of the reason, why is it that some individuals can eat less and lose a few pounds, while others develop an eating problem? In the field of eating disorders it is understood that genetics loads the gun and environment pulls the trigger. Individuals who are genetically predisposed to serotonin sensitivity are at a much higher risk to develop an eating disorder. Evidence suggests that altered brain serotonin function may contribute to traits seen in Anorexia Nervosa.[14]

When individuals restrict their intake, it affects the body in many ways. There are abnormalities in function in various parts of the brain and in certain brain circuits, as well as in a number of neurotransmitters, including serotonin and dopamine. As these changes occur, these individuals become more obsessed and begin to feel guilty about what they are eating and cut their intake back even more. Simultaneously, the body is slowing down digestion. They feel guilty about what they are eating and eat less because they now feel full with smaller amounts of food. The body and brain therefore become malnourished, as intake is restricted. As the eating disorder evolves, binging, purging, laxative use, compulsive exercise, and other ways to compensate for eating may develop.

THE USEFULNESS OF METABOLIC TESTING AND BODY COMPOSITION ANALYSIS

Despite being available since the 1980's, Body Composition Analysis has only recently been used with the eating disorder patient population. Treating eating disorder patients is complicated. The use of measuring body composition by Bioelectrical Impedance Analysis (BIA) shows the changes in the various body compartments (ie. lean weight and fat weight). The BIA also allows each patient to be used as their own control, allowing the clinician the ability to individualize their eating plan. It has been recognized as a simple and inexpensive instrument that can be used to differentiate between lean and fat tissues.[15] The combination of Metabolic Testing and Body Composition Analysis helps us identify malnutrition and make appropriate treatment recommendations based on the test results. Additionally, both tests are helpful motivating tools. The Body Composition Analysis is extremely useful in determining how malnourished the body is. The reactance level is an indicator of individuals who may be at high risk for re-feeding edema. This is a condition that occurs in individuals who are severely malnourished. Someone who experiences re-feeding edema is at a much higher risk for a cardiac event. This test also gives us an idea about how debilitating the disease has been and if the individual's body is one that is fairly resilient and compensates when it is starved or if the body uses vital tissue and needs aggressive nutritional support.

Both the Metabolic Testing and Body Composition Analysis are extremely helpful in convincing the individual and their family that starvation is affecting the body. Too often, if they do not "look sick" (e.g., have a low body weight), there is much denial from both the patient and/or the family. When faced with concrete data that shows the body is malnourished based on the test results, the patient and family are much more able to understand the severity of the illness. These two tests help convince even the most difficult patient that he or she is doing damage to the body and that they need to follow the recommendations to correct it. A typical reaction from a patient is, **"I didn't realize I was doing any damage to my body; I thought I was just being healthy."**

CHAPTER 2

The Eating Disorder Voice

"My life before treatment was quite literally a living hell. I mean it in a very real way. Every nagging obsessive thought and obsessive ritual I would go through in order to feel "OK", satisfactory, one more day fighting the "fat" demon. Every pulse of energy I had was willingly given to the dictates of the Eating Disorder. I hated doing this, but it was better than living fat (I am 5'4" and weighed less than 100 pounds). I can remember just waiting for night to come so I could sleep. It was the only time I had peace. The only time the voices quieted, and I did not have to feel being in the body I despised."

- Jeanette

THE EFFECTS OF A STARVING BRAIN

Individuals who are suffering from malnutrition begin to experience physiological and psychological changes that make them very vulnerable to an eating disorder. This chapter will further address how restricting food intake can ultimately lead to a change in brain chemistry, which results in an increase in anxiety, depression, and obsessive-compulsive thoughts. When individuals are severely restricting their food intake, they are in effect starving the brain. They also often feel unhappy and out of control. Restricting food is one concrete way to gain control and numb the pain.

Being preoccupied with food rules and rituals can also help reduce anxiety. Instead of thinking about things that they cannot control or change in life, thinking about *when* they are going to eat, *what* they are going to eat, and *when* they can exercise gives them a sense of control.

> "I don't know how it happened. I never thought about food and weight. Now I can't go through a day without preplanning everything I am going to eat, when I am going to exercise, checking out exactly what my mom is preparing for dinner, and double-checking the food labels. I try on at least five outfits every morning. I check and recheck myself in the mirror several times, wondering if I look fat. But maybe it's because I gained weight. I must have gotten fatter because I had to eat that potato last night. The only relief I get is when I finally can fall asleep".
>
> – Heather

HOW OBSESSIVE-COMPULSIVE THOUGHTS EVOLVE INTO THE EATING DISORDER VOICE

Imagine trying to eat and enjoy a meal when voices in your head are relentless and screaming thing like, ***"You're fat! Don't eat that! No one likes you! Your stomach is huge! You need to run more! You need to lose weight! You're a failure if you eat! Restrict, don't eat, be strong! You're not good enough!"***

The chaos and noise individuals with eating disorders hear is very harsh and critical, and this constant chatter is present any time they try to take a bite of food. This critical voice is their worst enemy. Professionals frequently refer to these obsessive thoughts as the *eating disorder voice*.

The obsessive-compulsive thinking, which initially happens a few times a day, will eventually consume most thoughts. This is a gradual process and most patients are unaware of the change until it has become all-consuming. The obsessive thoughts are typically about what foods they are "allowed" to eat, how much exercise they "must do," and "how weak they feel" if they don't follow "the rules."

"The eating disorder takes so much from the person to whom it attaches itself so ruthlessly, so slowly and desperately that the person may not even notice it. I became a shadow of my former self, but didn't realize that my once fun-loving and outgoing personality had withered into something more closely resembling a dull, bored, and often preoccupied shell. As a result, my social life withered, too. The scariest part of having an eating disorder was being stuck in it. In its all-consuming grip, it's all too easy to lose yourself entirely—without knowing you've lost anything more than weight."

–Nicole

BIOCHEMICAL CHANGES IN THE BRAIN WHEN THE BODY IS UNDERFED

How can someone who has never obsessed about food become worried about what is okay and not okay to eat? What happens in the brain that so dramatically changes how a person thinks about eating? When food intake is restricted either intentionally (e.g., on a diet) or unintentionally (e.g., from an illness), biochemical changes occur. The more restricted the intake is and the longer it lasts, the more it has an effect on the brain's chemistry. Eating less carbohydrates and protein will eventually affect how the brain circuits work and the level of neurotransmitters in the brain. Protein is broken down into the amino acid tryptophan. Tryptophan is a precursor needed to make serotonin and works with carbohydrates to cross the blood/brain barrier. This is needed to produce the neurotransmitter serotonin.[1]

Change in Brain Chemistry

When someone eats less, this affects the body's ability to produce neurotransmitters. This can lead to an increase in depression, anxiety, and obsessive-compulsive thoughts. Serotonin is also found in the stomach and plays a role in the body's slower emptying of the stomach. The slow emptying of the stomach (gastroparesis), combined with the increase in obsessive thoughts results in feeling guilty when eating. Eating less is one of the factors that leads to development of eating disorder.

"I thought I was just trying to eat healthier. I stopped eating sweets and ate less bread. I ate less because I felt full much sooner and felt guilty if I ate "unhealthy" foods. The less I ate, the less I wanted to eat. My stomach would feel full and heavy, even if I only ate a little. Any time I ate it felt like "I was pregnant.". My friends started to notice how little I was eating and tried to get me to eat more, but I thought they were overreacting. It wasn't until I went to the Nutrition Clinic that I realized I was actually doing damage to my body."

–Jill

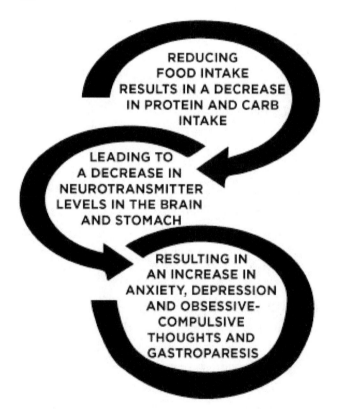

REDUCING FOOD INTAKE RESULTS IN A DECREASE IN PROTEIN AND CARB INTAKE

LEADING TO A DECREASE IN NEUROTRANSMITTER LEVELS IN THE BRAIN AND STOMACH

RESULTING IN AN INCREASE IN ANXIETY, DEPRESSION AND OBSESSIVE-COMPULSIVE THOUGHTS AND GASTROPARESIS

INCREASED OBSESSIVE-COMPULSIVE THOUGHTS

The less food individuals eat, the more obsessed they feel about what they should and should not eat. They begin to identify foods as "good and bad." Initially, they may feel guilty about eating "fattening foods," so fried foods, as well as fats and oils, are cut out. Carbohydrates are often restricted, such as bread, cereal, and other complex carbohydrates like potato, rice, and pasta are identified as "bad." Eventually, the "good" foods maybe limited to fruits, vegetables, and some lean protein sources.

At the same time, because the stomach is emptying more slowly (gastroparesis), they feel full with much less food and eat less because it feels uncomfortable to eat. Eventually, their bodies and brain become malnourished.

PSYCHOTROPIC MEDICATION

Food is the number-one thing the body needs. However, it can be very difficult to increase intake to an adequate level when the eating disorder voice is strong.

> *"I had to control so much of what I was eating just for the sake of "being healthy" that eating almost became a chore for me. I clearly remember having restless nights thinking about what I would eat the next day and how I could get through the day with the plan I laid out. I had to eat clean and exercise every day. I was so caught up in my day-to-day regimen. I wanted to be healthy, but my body and mind wouldn't allow it."*
>
> *–Soren*

If the patient is not able to increase intake because of the obsessive thoughts, psychotropic medication may help. The neurochemistry in the brain changes as a result of restricting food intake. Medication, such as antidepressants, may be used to help increase the neurotransmitters in the brain, which will aid in the recovery process.

> *"It wasn't until I agreed to try medication that the voices quieted down. Until then, every time I ate was such*

a chore. I would try to block [the voices] out, but they just got louder. When I finally agreed to try medication, I started to get relief. I could actually eat a meal and not obsess about it for the next two to three hours afterward!"

–Mary

A psychiatric evaluation is needed to determine if medication is appropriate. Some patients and/or the family are reluctant to use medication. A typical response is, "I want to do it naturally." It is important for the patient to understand that restricting intake is not natural and the amount of food intake needed to restore the brain chemistry can, in some cases, be difficult to achieve. Medication can help quiet the obsessive thoughts, reduce anxiety, decrease depression, and improve stomach function. In order for many psychotropic medications to be effective, the body needs to be nourished.[2] Metabolic Testing can identify individuals who may not have enough protein substrate available for medications to work.

WHY OBSESSIVE-COMPULSIVE THOUGHTS INCREASE WHEN NORMAL EATING RESUMES

We have often seen patients normalize their obsessive thoughts about food. They have become so accustomed to the *arguments* in their thoughts about food and weight that they do not recognize them as abnormal. When we initially evaluate a patient, it is a relief to them to realize that the thoughts are not normal and that with treatment they can decrease. It is also helpful for them to understand that the obsessive thoughts have been very purposeful. Instead of worrying about things they cannot change (e.g., marital problems their parents are having or getting a low grade on a test), they will start to obsess more about the food they eat, how much they weigh, and when they can exercise. This gives them something to focus on that they still feel they can control. We frequently see that it also helps them regulate their anxiety about the emotional issues they struggle with.

"Before I went to see Annika, I was constantly obsessing about food. I counted my calories every single day, yet I had no idea what my body actually needed. The only information I had was through the media, which told me

I needed 1,200 calories in order to maintain a thin frame. I was always hungry, but would barely let myself eat anything. I had cravings every day, which led to overeating some days, and restricting even more the following days. I was afraid to let myself skip a day of exercising, and had become compulsive about burning at least as much as I ate. Finally, I realized that I was flat-out unhappy. My usually bubbly self was always down, and it felt like I was constantly in a bad mood no matter how happy I wanted or tried to be."

– Jackie

As mentioned earlier, when food intake is reduced, a change in brain chemistry occurs and there is an increase in obsessive-compulsive thoughts. These thoughts help protect the person from feeling underlying uncomfortable feelings and emotional pain. But when food intake is increased, the "out of control" feelings will come back, and the eating disorder voice will fight the reemerging feelings of loss of control and pain. As an individual eats more, there is a change in brain chemistry, and initially their anxiety will be much higher. Patients often report that it feels worse before it gets better. Following a structured plan helps to decrease some of the anxiety. The repetition of a structured meal plan helps rewire the brain.[3]

"It was so difficult to trust that I had to eat. I had only eaten healthy and now they want me to eat so much more than I ever did! It was so helpful to not have any choice in what food I had to have. If I had to pick what I was going to eat, the eating disorder would take over. It was so exhausting to make any decision about food. It was such a relief to know exactly what I had to do and to keep repeating the same food at each meal. I eventually started to trust that I could vary my intake, but it came with a lot of practice before I was willing to trust that it would be okay."

– Mary

Eating an adequate amount of food is necessary for the brain to function properly. A starved brain cannot process the underlying emotional pain. As eating improves, it becomes easier to understand and benefit from the psychotherapy needed to address the underlying emotional pain. The goal is to normalize eating in order to minimize obsessive thoughts. This is a difficult process that takes food, therapeutic treatment and time, as well as patience.

To learn more about the eating disorder voice, go to Dr. Laura Hill's 2014 presentation at TEDX Columbus at http://www.scientificamerican.com/article/understanding-the-brain-may-help-explain-eating-disorders-video/.

CHAPTER 3

Metabolic Testing and Body Composition Analysis

"I was a little apprehensive going to my first visit, but the series of tests and concrete sets of numbers put forth gave me a sense of confidence in her expertise that I felt I was missing in other treatment facilities, and even at the offices of medical professionals. Being able to see how I was working internally was at first disconcerting, jarring, and literally unbelievable, starkly contrasting with information I had been given from other sources. But it was necessary and impossibly helpful in allowing me to see how I was functioning, and moreover, how I wasn't."

– Nicole

Metabolic Testing and Body Composition Analysis are two critical tests that have been a standard part of our practice. For over 20 years we have used them to test each and every patient that comes to us for treatment. These two tests are initially used as we prescreen our patients to provide us with a comprehensive nutritional assessment and see if they are malnourished. If patients are malnourished, we repeat the tests throughout treatment to measure and monitor their nutritional status. As described in the testimonial above, the testing helps a patient see first-hand how their body responds to their nutritional intake. It allows us to bring them into the conversation. In turn, they are more invested in their recovery.

When we initially meet with new patients, we do an extensive interview as part of the intake process. We are well aware that patients are not always as forthcoming about their eating disorder as they need to be, for a variety of reasons. Some may be too embarrassed to fully disclose their behaviors and symptoms, or they might be severely depressed and are unable to convey what they are experiencing. Other patients have become very adept at hiding the truth, especially if they are resistant to receiving help, and there are those who aren't aware their behaviors are unhealthy. Since we know that the complete picture of a patient's eating disorder cannot be revealed through an interview or the scale, we rely heavily on Metabolic Testing and Body Composition Analysis to provide us with a more accurate picture.

We firmly believe our high success rate in treating individuals with eating disorders comes from using these tests to measure health from within. Not only are we receiving information that provides us with the data needed for a thorough nutritional assessment, but we can also immediately determine the calories and nutrients needed for our patients to re-nourish their bodies and regain their health. Because a comprehensive nutritional assessment is the first step in the treatment of malnutrition, we need to have a complete history that takes into consideration food intake, body composition, resting metabolic rate, physical stressors, and medical, social, and family history, as well as exercise. Therefore, both tests are needed to accurately determine what is going on internally with our patients.

METABOLISM

To better understand Metabolic Testing, it is important to have a fundamental understanding of metabolism and the role it plays in whether or not a body is able to perform the necessary physiological functions. Food is need to provide the energy necessary to maintain life. Metabolism is the sum of the physical and chemical changes that occur in the body. Our body is working 24/7. Physical and chemical changes go on even during our sleep. We are forming new cells, hormones, enzymes, repairing tissue, growing bone and muscle, and many other processes that are all part of the metabolic functions.

Metabolism has two basic processes: anabolism and catabolism. Anabolism is the building-up of tissue; catabolism is the tearing down of tissue, or the body shrinking. For instance, if an individual is weight training, the goal is to increase muscle mass. If the body is adequately fed, anabolism will occur. However, if there is not enough fuel (food intake), the body will be catabolic (tearing down of tissue), which will result in less muscle mass.

Adolescents and teens are at a peak time in their life when the body should be building bone strength. When there isn't adequate food intake, the body is catabolic and has to use vital tissue (organs) to maintain itself. Instead of laying down bone, the body is using the bone to maintain the blood protein and calcium levels.

Our interest as health practitioners lies in the area of how metabolism is affected by eating disorders. We know that the body converts the food we eat into energy for the body to function. We also know that the body's basal metabolism represents the energy the body needs to maintain it's temperature, as well as the energy the organs need to function. What happens to an individual's metabolism when he or she has been restricting intake or purging? How has the body responded and how has it affected the metabolic rate? Knowing this information helps us see how resilient or at risk the body may be.

We have seen very different metabolic results, depending on the type of eating disorder behaviors the individual uses. For the individual that restricts calories, the body becomes hypometabolic and slows down to conserve the energy necessary for the daily functioning of the body. This individual may or may not be low body weight. Both anorexics and "high weight" anorexics will typically be hypometabolic.

Individuals who engage in bulimic behavior vary depending on the caloric value of the binge and the severity of the purging. Individuals that have high-calorie binges (1,000 calories or more) are usually normal or hypermetabolic. Individuals who restrict and purge are typically hypometabolic.

Individuals who struggle with compulsive overeating typically tend to restrict their calories early in the day and then overeat at night. This type of behavior usually results in the body slowing down or being hypometabolic. Binge-Eating Disorder patients vary based on the frequency of the binging and how they compensate for the binge. If they restrict through the day to compensate for binging and binge-eat at night, they are typically hypometabolic. If they binge throughout the day, they are usually hypermetabolic.

MEASURING METABOLIC RATE

To measure a patient's metabolism, we need to collect data that will determine a body's predicted resting energy expenditure (PREE). This data includes age, sex, and weight. The body's Actual Resting Energy Expenditure (AREE) is measured by Metabolic Testing. AREE is tested by measuring the body's oxygen and carbon dioxide exchange, or how much oxygen is consumed and carbon dioxide is produced at rest. The process is called indirect calorimetry.[1] Indirect calorimetry is the gold standard for measuring energy expenditure in a clinical setting. It is a scientifically based approach to customize a patient's energy needs and individualize the nutritional recommendations.[2] We use a computerized system for the collection, analysis, and output of the testing data.

Once the data is collected, we are able to see how a patient's body has responded to restricted calorie intake, purging, laxative use, compulsive exercise, binge eating, or compulsive eating. This helps us begin to understand how his or her body works and how it will respond to the re-feeding process. It also helps us determine how reliable the patient's information has been regarding the eating disorder behaviors.

How the Tests are Performed

As highlighted in the testimonial at the beginning of this chapter, many patients are apprehensive on their initial visits. However, we thoroughly explain the Metabolic Testing and Body Composition Analysis tests. Both procedures can be completed in less than 30 minutes.

To measure their ideal AREE, patients will come to the appointment after fasting for eight to 12 hours. They will also have abstained from any exercise during that period. However, if this is not possible, the following conditions should be met:

- No eating/drinking calories or caffeine four hours prior to the test.
- No exercise day of the test.
- No smoking two hours prior to the test.
- No stimulant medications two hours prior to test.

During the Metabolic Testing procedure, the patient sits in a reclining chair under a lightweight canopy hood. Reaching a steady state (when the breathing changes less than 10 percent) will typically take a few minutes. Once this is achieved, the test takes about 15 to 20 minutes. Patients are also given the Body Composition Analysis during the same visit. This test, which will be discussed in more depth below, is also noninvasive. It only requires the patient to lie down and have electrodes attached to the wrist and foot to pass a small electrical current through the body.

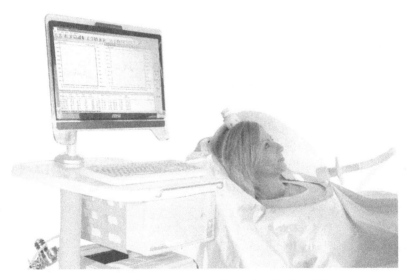

Figure 1: Metabolic Testing is a quick, noninvasive breathing test.

source: www.cosmed.it

METABOLIC TESTING: ANALYZING THE RESULTS

Of the several formulas used to calculate the amount of calories an individual should be burning, the Harris–Benedict Formula is commonly used.[3] This formula takes into consideration age, height, sex, and weight to determine the normal caloric expenditure for an individual. In addition to the AREE, an additional energy factor needs to be calculated. Light activity includes sitting, standing, working on a computer, etc., but no actual exercise. The energy expenditure of exercise, or how many calories are burned doing exercise, is also factored in.

Diagnosing Hypometabolic and Catabolic States

Metabolic Testing is critical to our treatment protocol because it allows us to quickly identify when a patient is malnourished and is in a hypometabolic and catabolic state. This test assesses if the body is burning the estimated calories it should be burning (normal metabolic), fewer calories than it should be burning (hypometabolic), or more calories than would be predicted (hypermetabolic).

If the patient is burning fewer calories than needed, this means the body's metabolism has slowed down. The hypometabolic state occurs when the body is not fed adequately, is stressed, and/or is trying to conserve energy. The body is trying to conserve the energy it needs for vital functions, so it down-regulates the metabolism. It also conserves energy by decreasing the body temperature, slowing down the heart rate, and no longer menstruating, among other means.

It is difficult for individuals to know if they are hypometabolic because the main symptom they have is feeling tired. However, being tired is not easily identified until their metabolism has improved and they start to feel better and have more energy. Their initial low level of energy is what they have become accustomed to, so that seems normal to them. Metabolic Testing allows us to identify any abnormalities and quickly devise a nutritional plan that best fits the clinical condition of the patient.

Metabolic Testing also measures the body's protein use—the amount of protein stores that are being used to help fuel the body. The body normally uses approximately 2 to 15 percent of its own protein stores to fuel the body. When more is being used, the body is breaking down its own lean tissue to fuel itself.[4] This is referred to as being catabolic. Catabolism is the breakdown of larger molecules into smaller units to release energy. When the body has not been sufficiently fed, it becomes catabolic and breaks down its own cells to use as energy.

A person is hypometabolic when the AREE is less than the PREE. This means the body is burning fewer calories than you would expect it to. The body is catabolic when the protein substrate use is more than 15 percent. This means the body is breaking down its protein tissue to use for energy to meet basic physiological needs. The hypometabolic/catabolic state occurs when the body's nutritional needs are not met and it has down-regulated the metabolism to conserve energy, using its own protein reserves (organ tissue, muscle, immune system) to maintain the physiological functions of the body.

Terry's Story

Terry was simply trying to eat healthier and lose weight. She decided to cut back on the amount of fat she was eating and eat less bread. Despite cutting back significantly on her intake, her weight remained the same. She came to the clinic to see why she couldn't lose weight. Her Metabolic Test showed she was severely hypometabolic, burning only 784 calories when she should be burning 1,321 calories at rest. It also showed that she was catabolic, using a significant amount of her protein stores; normally, the body breaks down approximately 15 percent or less of its protein stores, but she was using 37 percent. She was catabolic. Her body had down-regulated her metabolism to conserve energy because she was not eating enough to meet the body's needs.

Reaction to the Results

Metabolic Testing results can be extremely helpful in motivating a patient to make changes. The majority of individuals who struggle with eating disorders are in denial that they are doing any damage to their body. Their only gauge has been blood work, which is typically normal. If their body weight isn't low, then they don't think there is any physical problem. Any individual can be hypometabolic and catabolic, regardless of body weight.

Seeing actual results of tests that show how the body is functioning inside makes a difference. Educating the patient about how the body responds when it is underfed is something they have often heard, but seeing their own body responding in this way helps them begin to trust the treatment recommendations.

BODY COMPOSITION ANALYSIS

Body Composition Analysis (BCA), done by bioelectrical impedance, measures the composition of the body: that is, the amount of fat and lean tissue (lean dry mass or muscle, bone, organs, skin, hair, etc.) in the body. As with the Metabolic Test, BCA is also quick and noninvasive. Electrodes are attached to the wrist and foot of the individual and a small electrical current is passed through the body. BCA measures resistance and reactance to the current as it travels through water in lean tissue and fat. The test is based on the rate that the current passes through the cell and measures lean mass, body fat, lean dry mass (muscle), total body water, intracellular water, extracellular water, and phase angle.

Phase angle is a measurement based on total body resistance and reactance and is independent of height, weight, and body fat. A lower phase angle appears to be consistent with cell death or a breakdown of cell membrane and an inability of cells to store energy. A higher phase angle appears to be consistent with larger quantities of intact cell membranes and lean dry mass. A low phase angle is consistent with malnutrition, HIV/ AIDS, cancer, and chronic alcoholism. As the body is nutritionally restored, the overall cellular health of the individual improves, the cell membranes become more intact and the phase angle improves.[5] Phase angle is a predictor of outcome and indicates the course of disease.

> "During the first months of treatment I stubbornly argued with my treatment team, reasoning that my symptoms were not severe enough to constitute a real eating disorder. Although I was adept at rationalizing my disorder, when confronted with my body composition analysis at my weekly nutrition appointments it became difficult to maintain that my behaviors were innocuous. The numbers proved that they resulted in a consistent loss of lean body

mass. If that wasn't enough, a bone density test provided further evidence that I had wreaked havoc on my skeleton and a metabolic profile confirmed that I was severely hypometabolic. With the evidence before me, I had to admit that I was sick and needed help, I was harming my body."

– Julie

BCA is part of our treatment protocol. We use it as part of a case-management strategy and educate our patients on its results. We are aware that some patients may become obsessed with what their readings are going to be. These are typically patients who also weigh themselves multiple times per day. However, as they begin to understand how the body works and what fluid shifts feel like, they become more comfortable and less anxious.

"I was weighing myself several times a day before I came to the Nutrition Clinic. If I gained a pound I would eat less; if I stayed the same weight, I'd have to eat less; if I lost weight I would restrict to try and lose more. Not until I was able to understand the body composition analysis was I able to give up my obsessive weighing and trust my body."

– Jeanette

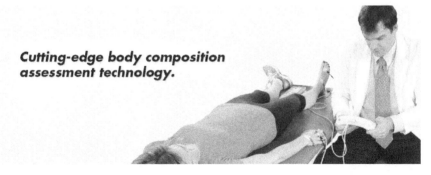

Figure 2: Body Composition Analysis by bioelectric impedance
source: rjlsystems.com

TAKING THE GUESSWORK OUT OF TREATMENT

> *"I didn't believe until the testing was done that I had seriously relapsed. My eating disorder had tricked me into believing that I was eating enough to fuel my body properly. When the test results were explained to me, it was very clear that my body was severely undernourished even though my body weight had changed very little."*
>
> *– Joslyn*

Metabolic Testing and Body Composition Analysis take the guesswork out of treatment. This becomes a helpful educational tool as patients go through the recovery process. Throughout this book, we will provide examples of how we actually employ the use of both tests when working with different eating disordered populations. These tests are underutilized but have the potential to revolutionize the treatment protocols for eating disorders.

Questions and Answers for Metabolic Testing and Body Composition Analysis

Q: How long will it take my metabolism to improve?

A: Your metabolism begins to improve as soon as you start to increase your caloric intake. The length of time depends on how severely hypometabolic you were, how much repair the body needs to do and if you are able to follow all the treatment recommendations. We have seen metabolic rates correct in six to eight weeks with total compliance and no exercise.

Q: Won't exercise improve my metabolism?

A: Exercise may actually slow your metabolism down. If you have been restricting your intake and over-exercising, your body has slowed down to conserve energy. Exercising when the body is trying to repair itself uses vital energy that the body needs to heal.

Q: If I eat more calories than my body is burning, won't I gain a lot of fat weight?

A: When the body is repairing, it is using the extra calories to restore the cellular integrity. The body will gradually weight restore both lean and fat weight. There may be initial weight gain but as the metabolic rate improves this stabilizes.

Q: How soon will you see changes in my Body Composition Analysis?

A: We monitor several changes with the Body Composition Analysis. Initially, we check for any fluid shifts that might indicate re-feeding edema. We also assess the changes in phase angle and lean dry mass. If there is a decrease in either one, the body needs more calories to improve.

Q: What is the difference between Body Composition Analysis and BMI?

A: BMI (Body Mass Index) measures the total body surface area, but does not take into account the body composition. Body Composition Analysis measures the composition of the body. This is why an athlete who has a large muscle mass can fall into the overweight or obese range according to the BMI, when he or she actually has a very little body fat. Body Composition Analysis is a much more accurate way to determine recommended body weight ranges.

Q: How can I be malnourished if I am weight restored?

A: Reaching your recommended body weight does not mean the body is burning a normal amount of calories and not breaking down protein reserves. You can be eating enough to gain weight, but not improve your metabolic rate. Using Metabolic Testing (indirect calorimetry) is the only way to determine if you have corrected your metabolic rate. The Body Composition Analysis measures phase angle, which helps us assess the body's cellular health.

Q: Will I be able to cut back on my intake once my metabolism has corrected?

A: The amount of calories you need is based on your body's resting energy expenditure needs plus the calories needed for your activity level. This will be determined by your dietitian/nutritionist.

CHAPTER 4

Anorexia Nervosa

"I was very fearful about getting help. It was difficult to change my ways and adopt a new way of doing things. I had become so used to restricting my intake, exercising excessively, having an empty stomach, being able to see my ribs, not being able to concentrate, falling asleep everywhere, not being able to do my work, and having people give me attention, that all this negativity became a form of comfort for me. I was a prisoner to a dangerous mindset and dangerous habits, but this prison was comfortable because it was all I knew. It was hard to increase my intake because I wasn't used to really nourishing my body in such a long time and I didn't want to gain weight."

– Colleen

DANGEROUS MINDSET, DANGEROUS HABITS

According to the *Diagnostic and Statistical Manual of Mental Disorders* (DSM-5), a person with Anorexia Nervosa has an intense fear of gaining weight, becoming fat, or has a persistent behavior that interferes with weight gain, even though he or she is at a significantly low weight. There is also an inability to judge or perceive one's body accurately, an over-evaluation of shape or weight, or difficulty recognizing the seriousness of the current low body weight. In addition, a person with Anorexia Nervosa often does not realize that he or she is "a prisoner to a dangerous mindset and danger-ous habits," as powerfully described in the patient testimonial above.

Anorexia Nervosa is characterized by food restriction leading to mal-nutrition and obsessive-compulsive thinking, causing a body weight that is substantially lower than normal or expected. Individuals who struggle with Anorexia Nervosa see themselves as being overweight, even when at an extremely low body weight. They typically weigh themselves repeatedly and are constantly thinking about food in an irrational way. The eating disorder voice is now part of their inner thoughts and is constantly letting them know there will be a consequence if they do not know, **"How many calories?" "How many fat grams?"** or **"How much do I need to exercise after I eat that?"** every time a bite of food is contemplated. The culmination is a dangerous mindset and dangerous habits. The death rate for Anorexia Nervosa in the U.S. is 12 times higher than for all other leading causes of death combined in the 15 to 24 age groups.[1]

THE IMAGE IN THE MIRROR

> *"I would look in a mirror hundreds of times a day. I would put my fingers around my wrist to make sure I hadn't gained any weight. I packed a scale in my backpack so I would weigh myself before and after each class. I was terrified that I was gaining weight."*
>
> *– Sara*

When anorexic individuals look into a mirror, they don't see an accurate reflection; instead, they see themselves as fat, even though they are sig-nificantly below minimal weight. This phenomenon is often referred to as "distorted body image" and results in continuous restricting. Along with non-stop restricting, anorexics also do body checks in a ritualistic manner. They are often weighing, measuring, pinching, or wrapping their hands around their stomach, waist, thighs, or arms.

The power of these body checks, coupled with the distorted image they see in the mirror, cannot be understated. The result is a forceful attempt to restrict their eating even more, not only because of the fear of gaining weight, but because the image in the mirror is becoming increasingly distorted. Rational thoughts regarding food become virtually nonexistent and meals are increasingly avoided or eaten very slowly. Each and every bite is pondered because there is fear that eating will surely add weight, especially fat, to the body. Severe food restriction leaves the body susceptible to a change in brain chemistry, as well as a hypometabolic and/or catabolic state and resulting in malnutrition.

IDENTIFYING ANOREXIA NERVOSA

Twenty four million Americans and 70 million individuals worldwide of all ages and gender suffer from an eating disorder.[2] According to statistics, 90 percent of all people with Anorexia Nervosa are female, with the majority being between the ages of 15 and 19. However, an increasing number of females 25 and older are also being diagnosed with Anorexia Nervosa. There is also a higher occurrence in males than in the past. These numbers result in eight to 11 million individuals who are afflicted with this eating disorder.[3] Twenty percent of people suffering from Anorexia Nervosa will prematurely die from complications related to their eating disorder, including suicide and heart problems.[4]

Because of the high incidences of this disease coupled with its high mortality rate, it is important for anyone who knows an individual (either personally or professionally) they suspect might be anorexic to be aware of the disorder's warning signs.

Warning Signs of Anorexia[5]
- Deliberate self-starvation
- Intense, persistent fear of gaining weight
- Refusal to eat or highly restrictive eating
- Excessive facial/body hair
- Compulsive exercise
- Abnormal weight loss
- Sensitivity to cold
- Absent or irregular menstruation in females
- Hair loss
- Body dysmorphia (negative thoughts about their body; believing they have a defect in either one or several features of their body)

Anorexics rarely self-refer themselves for treatment, so it is important for others in the community to do so. In our practices, we tend to receive referrals from clinicians, physicians, and other health practitioners, school personnel, and family members.

BEYOND THE WARNING SIGNS

Once a referral is made, we prescreen for physiological and psychological changes using tests, including Metabolic Testing and Body Composition Analysis, which go beyond the warning signs listed above.

Physiological Changes and Complications

Physiological changes and complications include the following:

Physiological changes. Even though severe weight loss is the most obvious symptom with anorexic patients, other physiological signs can range from gastric reflux to loss of muscle mass, heart palpitations, bradycardia (heart rate <60 beats per minute), and changes in brain functioning. Some symptoms are much more vague and can be misdiagnosed because they are characteristic of many different illnesses. These symptoms include weakness, fatigue, and dizziness due to low blood pressure (especially when going from sitting to standing)—all signs that the body is not compensating.

Stomach complaints. Feeling full, bloating, constipation, gastric reflux, and other general complaints such as **"I don't have any appetite,"** or **"if I eat I feel nauseated,"** are also prevalent symptoms. Gastroparesis can often be the cause of these types of complaints.

Other complaints. Dry skin, growth retardation, not growing the expected amount, insomnia, and poor sex drive are other complaints that need to be taken into consideration. Patients also may report chest pain, palpitations, or shortness of breath with any exertion.

Anorexia Nervosa is known to interfere with healthy skeletal growth, causing bone loss. Results from a 2014 study indicate that the development of Anorexia Nervosa markedly increased the risk of fractures during childhood and adolescence in girls with the disease when compared with those without a history of Anorexia Nervosa.[6]

Neurological and Psychological Changes and Complications

Neurological and psychological changes and complications include the following:

Neurological and psychological changes. Symptoms and changes in behaviors associated with Anorexia Nervosa include anxiety, irritability, depression, and emotional numbing. This happens when caloric intake is restricted, serotonin levels decrease, causing a change in brain chemistry. Cognitive symptoms include poor memory, poor concentration, low ambition, and lack of motivation. Psychological signals also include a pursuit of thinness, fear of gaining weight, denial of hunger, distorted body image, sense of ineffectiveness, isolation, and a struggle for control.[7] Other psychological risk factors may be a history of exposure to adverse events and circumstances and the presence of certain traits, such as perfectionism, obsessionality, social anxiety, shyness, excessive compliance, and low self-esteem.[8]

"Once I developed my eating disorder, I began to gradually seclude myself from my friends. The mere thought of going to their houses and eating their foods disturbed me. I saw them as barriers to my aspirations and as a result I didn't associate myself with them anymore. The only person who could ever truly understand me was

myself, so I thought. If anything, my time with Anorexia Nervosa was a time of idealization: a period where I believed I had the willpower to look like anything. It was absolutely unrealistic in every sense of the word, but I still felt like I could obtain the body of my dreams, almost like an object. In retrospect, it's disconcerting that I was willing to push myself that far for something that didn't exist."

– Soren

DENIAL IS PART OF THE DISEASE

One of the biggest obstacles to overcome when dealing with someone struggling with Anorexia Nervosa is the denial of the disorder. When adolescents and teens are referred for treatment, they are typically in denial and resistant to change. Metabolic Testing and Body Composition Analysis are very helpful in convincing the individual that they are doing harm to the body. In addition to low body weight, these tests are often the first findings that are abnormal. There is genuine inability on the patient's part to recognize the seriousness of the illness, in part because the initial intent was to "eat healthier and exercise." As the brain becomes starved, the ability to think rationally is impaired. This, combined with genuine fear of food, makes it very difficult for someone to eat. These tests take the guesswork out of what might be happening to the body and help convince them to eat.

CURRENT TRENDS IN ANOREXIA NERVOSA

Over the years, our practices have seen several changes in the food/exercise behaviors of the patient with Anorexia Nervosa. In the past, individuals with Anorexia Nervosa would severely restrict their calorie intake—a behavior that was relatively easy to identify. However, several changes in food behaviors have emerged in more recent years. More and more, we are seeing individuals who cut out fat intake, others who restrict carbohydrates or follow a gluten-free diet, and others who become vegetarian or vegan, hoping to avoid having to eat certain types of foods.

We are also seeing an increasing number of individuals eating only "healthy" foods—foods they consider to be "clean" foods or whole foods. This might sound very healthy to some, but when taken to an extreme can become very unhealthy. This is often referred to as Orthorexia Nervosa. When individuals are still eating what appears to be a healthy diet, it makes it much more difficult for the family to identify the eating disorder and also difficult for them to make a case for having the patient increase food intake. We are also starting to see an increase in two other cohorts requiring treatment for Anorexia Nervosa: post-bariatric (weight-loss surgery) patients, as well as children and pre-adolescents.

Anorexia Nervosa in the Bariatric Patient

Anorexia Nervosa and Bulimia Nervosa are difficult to identify in post-bariatric surgery patients. What starts out as restricting intake to lose weight can lead to severe restriction and starvation. These individuals are congratulated on their ability to lose the weight, but are not easily identified when it has been taken to an extreme.

> *"After my bypass surgery, I was thrilled with losing weight. My doctors were pleased with my weight loss and friends and family kept encouraging me to keep it up. I was terrified of letting people down. When I reached the weight I initially wanted to weigh, I wanted to lose more. I became obsessed about weighing myself several times a day and terrified I would start to gain. I ate less and less. My hair was falling out, but I didn't care; I only cared about the number on the scale."*
>
> *– Melissa*

The main mechanism bariatric surgery patients use to lose weight is eating less. The short-term results of bariatric surgery typically result in significant weight loss and an improvement in overall health.

Conditions such as Type 2 diabetes, high blood pressure, sleep apnea, and high cholesterol usually show initial improvement with weightloss, long term results are still being studied. Very specific dietary guidelines are recommended for post-bariatric patients. Eating problems can easily develop when these guidelines are not followed. Patients will describe involuntary vomiting when they eat too fast or eat certain foods. Some will learn to self-induce vomiting to alleviate the discomfort of overeating, some may eat to a point where they vomit involuntarily, and others may self-induce vomiting because of an eating disorder.

Despite a thorough evaluation prior to the surgery, eating problems can also develop after the surgery. Currently, a standardized assessment for post-operative eating behavior is lacking and new tools are needed to assess the changes that occur after surgery.[9] It is very difficult to identify those individuals who will develop eating problems post-op. What we do know is that multi-disciplinary treatment for all individuals pre- and post-op is highly recommended. Most of the individuals who we see in our practice did have an eating disorder history prior to surgery. However, they may not have been forthcoming with that information during the evaluation. This is a patient population that is very desperate to lose weight even at the expense of their long-term health.

Anorexia Nervosa at a Younger Age

In our practices, we are seeing an alarming increase of youth who are developing Anorexia Nervosa at a much younger age. Children and young adolescents are coming in already knowing what their Body Mass Indexes (BMI) are and wanting to tell us how much weight they need to lose. Anorexia Nervosa is hard to detect in children who are still growing because it may cause stunted growth, causing their height to be in proportion to their weight. Also, young children may not talk about losing weight, but rather describe physical complaints such as nausea or feelings of fullness—symptoms associated with other illnesses. Comments such as **"I can't eat that food, I'll get fat," "I don't want to weigh in the triple digits [100 pounds]," "I've never had anything but fat-free ice cream," "If I eat that I'll get a heart attack,"** and **"I won't have any friends if I don't lose weight,"** are becoming the norm from our younger patients.

This dialogue, combined with restricting their intake to get to a lower BMI, can spiral into an eating disorder for this younger cohort. It is important for any health-care practitioner dealing with the well-being of children and adolescents to understand the long-term consequences a well-intentioned comment such as, **"You just need to lose a few pounds,"** has on these young individuals.

> *"Our son had always been the smallest in his class. He was always on the low percentile at his yearly physical. When someone suggested he should be evaluated, we went along with it but assumed everything would be okay. His testing showed he was very malnourished. We tried to get him to eat more, but he always had an excuse: "I'm not hungry," "My stomach hurts," "I'll eat a little later," or "I ate before you got home." His bone density showed he was not developing his bones like he should; he was osteopenic. Eventually, he started to make comments like "I can't gain any weight because I won't run as fast." It was the first time he ever expressed the fears he had been struggling with for a long time."*

– Tyler's parents

What happens to the normal development of the brain when malnutrition occurs at an early age? Will these patients be more prone to depression, anxiety, and obsessive-compulsive disorder? Will it affect their brain's ability to function? These children may go undiagnosed if their body weight remains the same. It may take a few years for pediatricians to identify children who are not developing at a normal rate. Metabolic Testing and Body Composition Analysis help identify these individuals much sooner. Aggressive nutritional support is needed to decrease the long-term consequences of the eating disorder. This is much easier for parents to understand if they have testing that demonstrates the degree of malnutrition.

USEFULNESS OF METABOLIC TESTING AND BODY COMPOSITION ANALYSIS

The results of Metabolic Testing (MT) and Body Composition Analysis (BCA) provide concrete information and evidence that patients are malnourished and are doing damage to their body. When parents understand how the obsessive thoughts and the eating disorder voice have taken over their child's normal thought process, they are able to recognize the situation as an eating disorder and not something "they did wrong." The MT lets us know how many calories the body is burning, compared to what it should be burning when fully fueled. It also shows if the body is getting enough protein or if it needs to use its own lean tissue (muscle and organs) as expensive fuel.

> "We didn't realize the full extent of Anorexia Nervosa's toll on our daughter until she had the Metabolic Testing and Body Composition Analysis done. This helped convince our daughter that she needed to eat the quantities required to get better. Over the course of the treatment it was very difficult to maintain the caloric intake. As the month's passed, her metabolism was very stubborn and not improving. The metabolic profile provided convincing information to her (and us) that—while she continued to improve—she wasn't finished."
>
> – Allison's parents

In most cases of Anorexia Nervosa, the body has become hypometabolic and catabolic. The BCA measures fat tissue, lean tissue, and phase angle. Calories need to be increased until all are within normal range.

Patients need to understand they need to eat more, even when they don't feel hungry. The MT and the BCA have shown that the body is malnourished, causing the metabolism to slow down, which makes the individual feel less hungry and feel full much sooner. The body has also decreased its production of several enzymes needed to digest food. While being underfed, the body has taken energy (thousands of calories) from fat tissue, bones, organs, and nerves to make up for the deficit. By eating extra calories, patients will resume a normal metabolic rate. The body will get back to a balanced state. Their hunger signals will gradually return and guide the individual when and how much to eat to stay healthy. As they eat more, their body burns more calories.

Our patients tend to worry that their hunger seems to be increasing, even though they are eating more. We are then able to show them tests results that demonstrate their bodies are healing, and that their increased hunger is a sign that their metabolic rate is increasing.

Questions and Answers for Anorexia Nervosa

Q: What happens if I start eating and can't stop?

A: The body has an internal drive to restore its weight and it is not unusual to struggle with overeating or perceived binging. One of the biggest fears you might have is ***if I start to eat, I'm afraid I can't stop***. It is important to understand that the body has been robbed of calories because of restriction, excessive exercise, and/or purging for an extended period of time. In addition to weight restoration, the body is trying to repair cellular damage. As the body weight is restored and the cells are repaired, the desire to overeat will decrease. By consuming an adequate amount of carbohydrates, protein, and fat, the desire to overeat is decreased. The BCA is a way to measure the cellular repair in the healing process.

Q: How long does it take to correct my metabolism?

A: This depends on the resiliency of the body, the nutritional status of the body, and how chronic the condition has been. If you have been struggling with an eating disorder for several years, it will take longer to correct. It is necessary to follow the recommended caloric intake in order to correct the metabolic rate. A fairly resilient body may be able to correct in six to eight weeks. It has been our experience exercising will also slow down the body's ability to correct its metabolic rate.

Q: Why is it so hard to break "food rules (what's okay and/or not okay to eat)?"

A: Even though it may make sense that you need to eat more to get better, the obsessive thoughts will be telling you not to. Initially, the obsessive thoughts will be much stronger. As the serotonin level gradually increases, the obsessive thoughts will eventually decrease. Early on in treatment, distracting yourself at meals can help you get through this difficult time. Initially, the more repetitive the eating plan is, the less intense the obsessive thoughts will be.

Q: Why do I have to gain more weight if I am getting my menses?

A: You can menstruate and still be malnourished. The body weight needs to be restored to replete loss of bones, muscle, and fat. The BCA will guide us with healthy weight gain recommendations. The MT will determine when the metabolic rate is corrected.

Q: What are some changes I can expect as I increase my intake?

A: When you initially increase your intake, you may feel tired for one to two weeks then your energy will start to increase. You will also feel full and uncomfortable. As your metabolic rate increases, you will begin to feel hunger and the stomach function improves. If you feel the desire to overeat or binge, let your nutritionist know so your eating plan can be adjusted.

CHAPTER 5
Bulimia Nervosa

"I felt like I was living a double life. In my professional world I was accomplished and well respected. In my secret world all I thought about was binging, purging, and how disgusting I was. At 42 years old, I had accepted that my eating disorder would be with me all lifelong, skeptical that things could ever be better. I had hidden my disorder for more than 20 years from my friends and family. No one would ever guess I was making myself throw up three or four times every day."

– Louise

"I knew I needed help, but I didn't want to let my family down. I was always the daughter they were proud of. I did well in school, was a top athlete, had several friends, but had this horrible secret. How could I ever tell them I was making myself throw up? I didn't want them to be ashamed of me."

– Alice

EXPOSING THE SECRETS OF BULIMIA NERVOSA

Bulimia Nervosa is derived from the Greek word meaning "ravenous hunger." Bulimia Nervosa is characterized by recurrent episodes of binge eating, defined as the consumption of a very large amount of food in a relatively short period of time, and associated with a perceived loss of control (not able to prevent or stop the behavior). This is coupled with regular compensatory behaviors (often referred to as purging) that are intended to prevent weight gain, such as self-induced vomiting, fasting, excessive exercise, and misuse of laxatives, diuretics, or other medications. The binge eating and purging both occur, on average, at least once a week for three months. The person's self-evaluation is unduly influenced by body shape and weight.[1]

Bulimia Nervosa is often a very secretive disorder, and many of those struggling with Bulimia Nervosa may feel they have failed at being anorexic. They would love to be able to restrict and not purge, but often their hunger and cravings take over, resulting in a binge. It has been our experience that what initially begins as restricting intake can easily spiral into Bulimia Nervosa. This happens for a variety of reasons. These individuals may be hungry and overeat or binge, feeling immediate remorse and have to "get rid of it" by self-induced vomiting, laxative, or diuretic use, or exercising to compensate. They may also be frustrated because despite severely restricting their intake, they are no longer losing weight.

THE FALLOUT FROM PURGING

Many people with Bulimia Nervosa initially begin to purge, hoping they will be able to lose more weight. In addition, many will purge any time they are emotionally upset, regardless of how little they have eaten. They describe the purging as a way to reduce their anxiety. The intensity of the purge (how many times they make themselves vomit) can put them at higher risk for fluid and electrolyte imbalance.[2]

Similar to people with Anorexia Nervosa, it is important for the person with Bulimia Nervosa to understand that binge eating and purging are behaviors used instead of expressing how they feel and what they need. They are very quick to dismiss their needs, and their self-talk can be very critical, negative, and unpleasant. Binge eating and/or purging will temporarily make them feel numb. However, the toll purging takes on the body is significant—the fallout can cause complications in the body that are quite harmful and damaging. Not only is the body trying to cope with the effects of malnutrition, but also the harsh effects of purging then heighten these complications.

Vomiting can cause severe gastrointestinal reflux symptoms, including heartburn, spontaneous vomiting, and acid regurgitation. Gastrointestinal symptoms due to vomiting and purging in absence of significant weight loss can resolve fairly quickly compared to those individuals with significant weight loss.

The throat area can also be harshly affected, as purging causes inflamed vocal cords, dysphagia (difficulty swallowing), laryngitis, and a high frequency of sore throats. Bulimics who purge through vomiting are also at a high risk for Mallory Weiss esophageal tear. Individuals who use ipecac to induce vomiting are at risk for irreversible cardiomyopathy (damage to the heart muscle), even after the Bulimia Nervosa subsides.[3]

For those who use laxatives, rebound constipation and fluid retention can develop as the bowel becomes dependent on laxatives. Laxative use is an ineffective means of weight loss; the weight change is loss of fluid.[4]

Compulsive exercising is another form of purging and is a strategy used by an overwhelming number of bulimics. Studies show that more than 90 percent of them exercise to compensate for binge eating and to make them feel better about their bulimic behavior. This will be discussed more in depth in chapter seven.

PRESCREENING, DIAGNOSING, AND TREATING BULIMIA NERVOSA

Bulimia Nervosa has many physical consequences, but it is important to note that bulimics can look healthy. They are often very ashamed of their behaviors and struggle disclosing them. When prescreening, diagnosing, or treating patients with Bulimia Nervosa, clinicians need to continually ask them which behaviors they are engaging in and the frequency. Individuals who struggle with Bulimia Nervosa often change their symptoms frequently. They may say they are doing much better because they have not purged in five days, yet their calorie intake is still severely restricted.

Individuals diagnosed with Bulimia Nervosa also describe binging very differently than those who binge as a result of other eating disorders. To some, eating "one more bite than I should" or eating more than they feel they should eat at a meal can also be perceived as a binge. A typical binge is eating an amount of food that is definitely larger than what most individuals would eat in a similar period of time under similar circumstances. It is much more important to evaluate the patient's symptoms than which diagnosis they may fall under.

WARNING SIGNS OF BULIMIA NERVOSA[5]

- Evidence of binge eating, such as the disappearance of large amounts of food in short periods of time, or the presence of wrappers and containers indicating overeating.
- Evidence of purging behaviors, including frequent trips to the bathroom after meals, signs and/or smells of vomiting, presence of wrappers or packages of laxatives or diuretics.
- Excessive, rigid exercise regimen—despite weather, fatigue, illness, or injury, the need to "burn off" calories taken in.
- Unusual swelling of the parotid glands (the cheeks and/ or jaw area).
- Calluses on the back of the hands and knuckles from self-induced vomiting.
- Discolored or stained teeth.
- Creation of lifestyle schedules or rituals to make time for binge-and-purge sessions.
- Withdrawal from usual friends and activities.
- In general, behaviors and attitudes indicating that weight loss, dieting, and control of food are becoming primary concerns.

BEYOND THE WARNING SIGNS

The following physiological and psychological changes and complications are often associated with Bulimia Nervosa. Many of the complications have to do with the effects purging has on the body, as well as malnutrition. Many patients in this population have physiological changes and complications.

Physiological Changes and Complications

Physiological changes and complications include the following:

Common complaints. Common complaints include cramping, diarrhea, esophagitis, inflamed vocal cords, and ulcers. Laxative use causes damage to the intestines and can often result in long-term dependency on laxatives for "normal" bowel movements. This damage to the intestine may take years to repair and sometimes never fully repairs. Diuretics can cause kidney damage and long-term blood pressure problems.[6] Other common complaints include swollen salivary glands (parotid glands, in particular). Dental erosion and increased dental sensitivity to cold or hot temperatures are common, as well as increased risk of dental caries. Dentists are often the first to identify the bulimic patient. Dental problems can occur long after the purging has ceased.[7]

Cardiac complications. Self-induced vomiting can result in low potassium levels causing heart irregularity. The risk of a cardiac arrhythmia due to a low potassium level will be much higher with an individual that is purging six to eight times a day.[8]

Neurological and Psychological Changes and Complications

This population also displays signs of other types of impulsivity. In addition to binging/purging, they are also at high risk for binge drinking, reckless overspending, shoplifting, and promiscuity.

Serotonin and dopamine levels. Individuals who do not have an eating disorder get an increase in dopamine when they enjoy the foods they are eating, as dopamine stimulates the pleasure and reward centers of the brain. However, Bulimics get less pleasure from food as it can be dull and tasteless.[9]

Mood instability and anxiety. Individuals who struggle with Bulimia Nervosa typically suffer from extreme mood changes and a high level of anxiety.

Suicide risk. A study headed by Sonja Swanson through the National Institute of Mental Health in 2011 found that among adolescents aged 13 to 18 who struggle with Bulimia Nervosa, 50 percent had thoughts and/or plans of suicide and 35 percent had actually had one attempt.[10]

Distorted body perception. Individuals struggling with Bulimia Nervosa have a very distorted perception of their body.

Carol's Story

The following is a case study of a female patient struggling with Bulimia Nervosa. The test results show how her body responded to a restricted intake and purging.

Carol is a 21-year-old who was diagnosed with Type 1 diabetes at age 16. She always had difficulty regulating her weight. Shortly after being diagnosed with diabetes, she began to struggle with Bulimia Nervosa. She was aware of the dangers of withholding her insulin, but was also fearful of having low blood sugar reactions. As a result, she would not use an adequate amount of insulin.

Carol continued to struggle with her weight and gained about 30 pounds in a year. Her Metabolic Test showed that she was severely hypometabolic. She was an athlete and should have been burning approximately 2,400 calories a day; she was only burning 845 calories. She was also catabolic; her protein substrate utilization was 30 percent, with normal being 15 percent. She was working out 90 minutes a day to get in shape for soccer season.

She had not been pleased with her training gains. Despite lifting weights for four months, she had not increased in strength. She felt tired all the time, but was working two jobs and thought this was normal. She would typically follow a restricted intake during the day, but by nighttime she was hungry and would binge on bread, cereal, and desserts and then purge. She struggled with a high level of depression and anxiety. She had been on medication but didn't think it helped, so she discontinued it.

The Metabolic Test results were very helpful in motivating Carol to make changes. She was a nutrition major and tried to eat only healthy foods, except when she struggled with binging. She didn't believe she needed to eat 2,500 calories a day despite her level of activity. She was willing to follow the recommendations because she knew we would be using the results of the Body Composition Analysis to guide us.

Over the first few weeks of treatment, she gained weight but felt much better. She was able to concentrate and focus and her energy significantly improved. After the initial weight gain, her body stabilized and she then began to decrease her fat weight. At the same time, she increased her calories to meet her body's needs. Over the course of three months, she increased her muscle mass by seven pounds.

She also agreed to go back on medication. When she was initially put on it, she was hypometabolic and catabolic; there was little substrate for the medication to work. Now that she was eating, Carol had a much better response to the medication. Throughout the whole treatment course, she experienced three pounds of overall weight gain. Her diabetes was much better managed and she could not believe how much better she felt.

THE USEFULNESS OF METABOLIC TESTING
AND BODY COMPOSITION ANALYSIS

> *"The initial evaluation was a wake-up call. My blood work was always normal despite the fact I might purge as many as six to ten times a day. The Metabolic Test showed how few calories I was burning and that I was using my own lean tissue, not fat, to exist. This was the first test that ever indicated that there was something wrong."*
>
> *– Jen*

It is not unusual for an individual to be very symptomatic with binge/purge behaviors and still have normal blood work. It is amazing how some bodies compensate. Since we are looking to measure our patients' health from within, we rely on Metabolic Testing to nutritionally assess them and determine whether or not they are hypometabolic and catabolic. Additionally, the Body Composition Analysis is very helpful in evaluating individuals with Bulimia Nervosa because it can be used to assess cell integrity (seeing how healthy an individual is at the cellular level) and showing if there has been a significant decrease in fat-free mass or muscle, despite weight being within normal range. Individuals who are symptomatic from binging/purging are typically very dehydrated. Many of the purging behaviors—self-induced vomiting, laxative use, and diuretic use—affect the hydration status of the body. The BCA measurements can also help identify those individuals who may be at high risk for re-feeding edema.[11]

Ongoing BCA helps identify individuals who are struggling with symptoms such as binging, purging, laxative or diuretic use, and compulsive exercise. This can be very helpful because people with Bulimia Nervosa often struggle with shame about the behaviors they engage in. Knowing that the test results indicate symptoms, helps them be more forthcoming with how much they have been binging or purging. Metabolic Testing and Body Composition Analysis usually helps motivate our patients, resulting in them following treatment recommendations when they are able to see what is happening to their body with the actual test results.

Questions and Answers for Bulimia Nervosa

Q: What can I change to decrease my desire to binge?

A: The desire to binge can be caused by underlying emotional issues, a physiological state, or a combination of the two. To decrease the body's physiological drive to binge, it will help to eat one-third of your recommended calories and protein intake at breakfast and another third by mid-afternoon. Mouth hunger and sweet cravings are signs that protein intake is inadequate. Balancing your food intake will decrease the physiological drive to binge and allow you to begin to work on the emotional triggers for binging.

Q: What can I do to avoid purging?

A: There are also many psychological reasons why individuals purge. Physical triggers, such as the stomach feeling heavy, often result in a purge. We have found using gastric digestive enzymes when you eat will decrease the heaviness in the stomach. Work with your therapist and dietitian/nutritionist to develop strategies to decrease your desire to purge. Tools like journaling or a mindfulness activity to decrease anxiety can be helpful.

Q: Why is my blood work normal despite how frequently I purge?

A: The body compensates in many different ways to maintain normal blood levels. It draws from your body's reserves such as bone to maintain balance. Simply because your blood work might be normal one day does not mean that it can't fall to a dangerous level in a short time period.

Q: Why does my weight fluctuate so much when I try to start eating and not purge?

A: Your body has become used to being dehydrated. It will hold on to fluid if you are someone who has been symptomatic with binging and purging. Gradually, as the body becomes more hydrated, the fluid shifts will be much less. Rapid changes in weight are related to fluid changes. If you notice your legs and feet are swollen, contact your doctor immediately. This may be a sign of re-feeding edema.

Q: If I am purging everything I eat, why can't I lose weight?

A: The body absorbs up to 50 percent of the calories you consume regardless if you purge. Even when very symptomatic, the body will hold at least 1,200 calories to fuel itself.

Q: Is there anything I can do to relieve the heavy stomach that I feel shortly after I eat even a small amount?

A: You are probably suffering from gastroparesis (a slow moving gut). We have found that a multi-enzyme formula or gastric digestive enzymes can help relieve this until the body's enzyme production has normalized.

CHAPTER 6

Binge Eating Disorder

"I just can't stop myself. I can't wait for my drive home. I stop at three different fast food places and order as much as I can without feeling embarrassed. I don't stop eating until I feel so full I can't eat any more. It's the only way I can feel relaxed before I have to face the chaos at home."

– Patricia

"I am so fearful of going to see my doctor. Every visit I get a lecture about how unhealthy it is to be overweight and how much better I would feel if I would just try to lose weight. I would never tell him I binge every day and that I do it even more when I know I have to go and see him. Of course I know I would be better off if I could lose weight, but I just can't stop myself!"

– Karen

I JUST CAN'T STOP MYSELF

Individuals struggling with binge eating often feel tremendous shame and have great difficulty talking about their relationship with food. They deny themselves certain foods and feel they do not deserve to eat what their body actually wants and/or needs. They feel like a failure because they lack willpower to control their food behaviors. Despite being aware of the health risks associated with binge eating, they cannot stop themselves, but would love to have a normal relationship with food.

Binge Eating Disorder (BED) is often unrecognized, misdiagnosed, or misunderstood by professionals, but it is actually *the* most prevalent of all eating disorders. Many who want to control and lose weight are just told to eat less. This over-simplified solution fails to recognize the underlying problems and feelings of helplessness that often accompany this disorder.

The DSM-5 defines binge eating as "recurring episodes of eating significantly more food in a short period of time than most people would eat under circumstances, with episodes marked by feelings of lack of control." When treating patients who are part of this population, we often hear frustration and embarrassment as they describe how they often eat quickly and do not stop when full. "I just can't stop myself" is often accompanied by tremendous shame.

WHY DOES SOMEONE BINGE?

Binge eating often starts out at a very young age. In this patient population, binging is often brought about because of emotional reasons. Many individuals diagnosed with a Binge Eating Disorder (BED) did not have their emotional needs met while they were growing up. They turned to food—a companion that was always there, did not judge, and would not be taken away. Food helped fill a void when nothing else was available. Binge eating is a behavior that often goes undetected, and therefore undiagnosed, unless there is significant weight gain. Families and medical providers would be concerned about the health of the overweight child, not realizing there were emotional reasons why they engaged in this behavior.

To the individual struggling with BED, the eating disorder voice has always been there. Comments like, **"I can't believe how disgusting you are," "You don't deserve to be eating that," "Why would anyone care about you," "You are just fat and lazy,"** and **"You'd be thinner if you just had some willpower,"** play over and over in their thoughts.

Dieting can also trigger BED in individuals in their teen or adult years, who have been struggling with constant dieting and weight cycling. Each time they restrict their intake, the neurotransmitter levels in the brain are adversely affected. If diets are short-term there is less of an effect, but if they are long-term or if the individual is following a very low-carbohydrate diet, the result is a significant increase in obsessive thoughts and the eating disorder voice. As they continue to restrict their intake, they are able to "do good" early in the day and then over-eat or binge in the evening. This is another pattern that sets patients up to struggle with BED. This unbalanced intake typically leads to increased hunger by midday and insatiable hunger at night, resulting in binge eating and starting a vicious cycle that is difficult to stop. Individuals who exercise at a high level but don't adequately fuel themselves are also at risk to struggle with binging.

Binge eating, or what is perceived as it, can also be a physiological response from Anorexia Nervosa. When the body has been starved, increased hunger is the body's normal response, because it needs fuel to repair its cells. This might create a strong desire to overeat or binge. Eating more allows the body to repair at its own pace, and the hunger will eventually decrease as the body's needs are met. Individuals also numb emotional pain and address unmet needs, anxiety, and/or stress by binge eating. There is a high incidence of binge eating when a person is in extreme emotional pain, causing them to dissociate (although physically present, the person is at times detached from reality). Individuals struggling with this type of binge eating are not always aware of what or how much they ate. The only way they know they binged is that there are food wrappers or empty containers left.

IDENTIFYING BINGE EATING DISORDER

"I don't understand it! I can be healthy for three or four days and then eat everything I can get my hands on for the next couple of days."

– Joan

BED is the most prevalent of all eating disorders. Since it is so prevalent in our society, it is important to understand the causes and risk factors, its warning signs, and the health consequences of this disorder. Unlike individuals with Anorexia Nervosa, binge eaters tend to be self-referrals. However, they are typically seeking help for weight loss and then are diagnosed as binge eaters. Referrals for children and teens often come from concerned family members and their primary care physician, but once again, they are referring for weight reasons, unaware there is an actual eating disorder.

WARNING SIGNS OF BINGE EATING DISORDER[1]
- Eating larger than normal amounts of food
- Eating even if full or not hungry
- Eating rapidly during binge episodes
- Eating until being uncomfortably full
- Feeling that the eating behavior is out of control
- Feeling disgusted, ashamed, or guilty about eating too much
- Experiencing depression and anxiety
- Feeling isolated and having difficulty talking about feelings
- Frequent dieting
- Losing and gaining weight repeatedly, also called yo-yo dieting

BEYOND THE WARNING SIGNS
Physiological and psychological changes and complications are associated with BED.

Physiological Changes and Complications
Individuals who struggle with BED may also struggle with obesity and weight gain. Other complications that might arise associated with obesity and weight gain are high cholesterol, Type 2 diabetes, hypertension, and heart disease. Other complications due to weight gain may include joint pain and arthritis.

These complications may be because of the binging and weight gain or can also be caused from weight cycling or yo-yo dieting. Weight gain often occurs with binging because of the types of foods consumed (high sugar and fat content). Periods of binging may be followed by a very restricted intake to compensate for the binge. It is the under/over eating pattern that causes the body to be hypometabolic and more susceptible to weight gain.

Neurological and Psychological Changes and Complications
Individuals who struggle with BED are often very self-conscious and ashamed of their physical appearance. They suffer from depression,

loneliness, and isolation. They tend to avoid activities centered around food and will binge in isolation. They tend to be very self-loathing and are very sensitive to comments about weight or appearance. Anxiety levels are usually very high and the binging helps decrease this. Individuals with BED often dissociate, typically during a binge.[2] They often struggle with concentration and focus because of their preoccupation with food.

THE USEFULNESS OF METABOLIC TESTING AND BODY COMPOSITION ANALYSIS

Terry's Story

Terry's story is an excellent example of the value of Metabolic Testing and Body Composition Analysis in helping someone struggling with BED.

Terry, a 29-year-old female, came in for treatment because she was gaining weight. At 5'4" her normal weight was 120 to 123 pounds, but over the past three years she had gained 20 pounds. As a fitness instructor, she exercised one to two hours a day. To lose weight, Terry had increased the time spent exercising to three hours a day. Metabolic Testing showed her being hypometabolic, burning only 1,108 calories per day when predicted was 2205 calories. She was also catabolic with a protein turn-over of 32% normal being 15%, using an excessive amount of her own lean tissue for energy. Terry ate 1,200 calories per day but struggled with binge eating five to six times a week, usually in the evening. A typical binge consisted of consuming approximately 1000 to 3000 calories. She was able to "be good" during the day and then struggled at night. After binging, the next day she would try to restrict her intake even more, but would eventually binge.

Terry's metabolism had slowed down because she was restricting her intake early in the day and then over-eating at night. She had also increased her exercise without increasing her caloric intake, which resulted in an even lower metabolic rate as the body tried to protect itself from starvation.

Terry was relieved when told to reduce her exercise level to only 30 to 45 minutes of cardio five days a week and to increase her intake to 1,800 to 2200 calories a day. She initially gained five pounds, the majority of it muscle. Her metabolic rate increased and was back to normal within three months, which is when she began to lose weight. By eating more, her binge eating episodes decreased and she realized that the only time she would struggle with binge eating was when she had skipped breakfast. Her energy level increased dramatically, she was much more satisfied with meals, the obsessive thoughts decreased, and her mood improved. Without the Metabolic Testing, Terry would have never believed she was malnourished and needed to increase her calorie intake to decrease her binging.

Metabolic Testing and Body Composition Analysis have proven to be invaluable tools in our practices when prescreening, diagnosing, and treating patients who have a Binge Eating Disorder. The case study above is an example of how we employ Metabolic Testing for someone with BED. Initially, we use it to identify whether or not malnutrition is present and if patients are hypometabolic. When individuals struggle with BED, they often binge at night and then restrict during the day to compensate. This under/over eating pattern often results in a slower metabolism. Because the body is not burning enough calories, they will gain weight. Increasing the caloric intake earlier in the day helps increase the metabolism.

These individuals also fall victim to believing that eating more than 1,200 calories a day is over-eating. We use the results from both tests to educate patients about their bodies. This convinces them in the long run that it is okay to increase their intake. Body Composition Analysis is also very helpful in determining an adequate eating plan for the BED patient.

Typically, these individuals have a larger lean mass and need more calories and protein to sustain it. An appropriate eating plan can be tailored to meet their needs based on the Body Composition Analysis results. The majority of binge eaters typically restrict their intake earlier in the day, which leads to binging later at night. It is commonly the imbalance of their calorie intake that sets them up to binge. Front-loading the calories of the day and increasing the protein intake can significantly decrease the frequency of binging.

TREATMENT PROTOCOLS FOR BED

Treatment for all patients with BED begins with an attempt to balance their intake in order to determine if their binging is related to physiological reasons. It is important to factor out this type of binge behavior to help identify patients who are emotional binge eaters. Some binge eaters simply need to balance their intake. This, however, is not the majority of those who struggle. Balancing out the intake gives the binge eater a sense of control and will typically decrease the initial binging, but they will soon return to their normal patterns because the reason they binge is usually more psychological than physiological.

In both of our practices, we find it very rewarding to work with this patient population. Their reaction to the initial assessment is one of great relief. They assume they are going to be handed another diet and told what they should not be eating. Instead, they are active players in their recovery; they are taught what their body needs and the test results reinforce when their bodies are malnourished or beginning to thrive. While we want patients to have a better understanding of their bodies, we do not include weight loss as a focus of the treatment protocol since this can be very damaging to the process of recovery. Recovery is much more than making changes in food and exercise behaviors; it is about working with the relationship patients have with food and exercise, and understanding any underlying emotions that they attach to them.

Questions and Answers for Binge Eating Disorder

Q: What are the causes of binge eating?

A: There are many different reasons for binge eating, some of which could be physiological, emotional, and/or sociocultural. This explains why it is so important to have a treatment team including a physician, therapist, and nutritionist to help the patient address binge eating. Without balancing nutritional intake, it is impossible to treat the Binge Eating Disorder.

Q: What is the difference between binge eating and compulsive overeating?

A: Compulsive overeating is eating in conjunction with a distracted activity such as watching television or studying. Individuals often do this when they are anxious. It is not the quantity or type of food, but the combination of being distracted and eating that calms them down. Binge eating is eating a large amount of food very rapidly. Typically, a binge can range from 500 to 2,000+ calories.

Q: Are there ways to change my food intake to decrease or stop binge eating?

A: Yes, first and foremost, stop dieting; develop an eating plan with a nutritionist that is realistic and healthy.

Q: How often should I eat?

A: Eat breakfast and continue to eat something every three to four hours. Make sure to have an adequate amount of protein with each meal and snack. Establish a regular eating pattern; eat at least one-third of the total daily caloric intake by noon and another one-third by 3:00 to 4:00 p.m. This means that if someone is on a 1,800-calorie diet with 80 to 100 grams of protein per day, breakfast should have approximately 600 calories with 25 to 35 grams protein. When intake is balanced, the desire to binge will decrease because of increased satiety throughout the day.

Q: What should I do if I have mouth hunger or food cravings?

A: When struggling with any type of binge eating, it is important to make sure the body is adequately fed. If the body is nutritionally out of balance, the individual will experience mouth hunger and food cravings, which increase the risk of binge eating. Mouth hunger is when the individual is not physically hungry, but wants something to eat. It can even occur shortly after finishing a meal, because of lack of satiety.

Q: Do you recommend therapy?

A: Definitely. It is difficult for binge eaters to discuss their behaviors with anyone. The judgment and shame they feel in the doctor's office can be very real, stopping them from asking for the help they so badly need. Since there are underlying emotions that are part of binge eating, we highly recommend working with caring and understanding professionals, including therapists or counselors, and letting family members or close friends take part in the treatment to help support the road to recovery.

CHAPTER 7

Compulsive Exercise

"I know I am going to be traveling this week for work. I can't let it get in the way of my exercise schedule. If I get up at 4:30 a.m., I can do my crunches and then go to the fitness center at the hotel. I can get there right when it opens so I can get a treadmill, run for 60 minutes and then do the stepper for 30 minutes. What happens if I can't get the treadmill? I could eat less, but I have to do my exercise in the morning. It can't wait till later in the day. Maybe I should just cancel my trip."

– Jerri

WHEN ENDORPHINS MEET THE EATING DISORDER VOICE

Endorphins are responsible for what is known as runner's high, the euphoric feeling a person receives from intense physical exercise. When individuals exercise, their levels of circulating endorphins and serotonin levels increase. These levels are known to stay elevated for several days after an exercise session, possibly contributing to improvement in mood and weight management. Moderate exercise can also improve mental health; it helps prevent depression, enhances or maintains positive self-esteem, and can even augment an individual's body image. The proven benefits exercise has on the body often results in healthcare providers calling it the "miracle" or "wonder" drug.

But what happens when exercise co-occurs with an eating disorder? Does exercise cease to become a miracle drug and instead becomes something to be avoided because of its addictive qualities? Do the positive effects of exercise become diminished or extinguished by the eating disorder? What happens to these endorphins and serotonin levels that circulate throughout the body once exercise becomes addictive? These are questions that interest us as practitioners. The patient who wrote the testimonial above most likely started to exercise to be healthier. But as this testimonial demonstrates, the eating disorder voice certainly has the ability to overpower any of the positive mental effects endorphins can have on the body and quickly eradicates any positive effects that might be derived from exercise.

GIVING COMPULSIVE EXERCISE THE ATTENTION IT DESERVES

The DSM-5 does not diagnose compulsive exercise as a separate eating disorder and instead includes it under Bulimia Nervosa. Because compulsive exercise affects so many eating disordered individuals and is one of the most difficult behaviors to treat, we feel it is important to discuss it independently. Studies have shown that high levels of exercise predict longer periods/duration of eating disorder hospitalization[1], and patients struggling with Anorexia Nervosa are quicker to relapse when resuming exercise within the first three months following discharge.[2] Studies also show that more than 90 percent of people with Bulimia Nervosa exercise to compensate for binge eating in order to make them feel better about their bulimic behavior.[3]

Compulsive exercise often serves to alleviate feelings of anxiety and guilt, whether or not they are related to eating. It can also serve to cover up uncomfortable feelings that are creeping up. Exercising provides individuals with the permission they need to eat or to make up for an earlier binge, or can be used as a way to control or manipulate their bodies to reach a certain weight goal. As nutritionists, we are concerned about the nutritional status of the disordered eater who does not fuel the body adequately for their level of activity—this can easily lead to malnutrition.

IDENTIFYING COMPULSIVE EXERCISE

Individuals who struggle with compulsive exercise may be difficult to identify initially. Yes, there are those individuals in which it is very obvious—they exercise three to four hours per day while severely restricting their intake. But there are also those who appear to be using activity in moderation. In this patient population, it is much more the attitude toward the activity than the amount of exercise. Listening to patients' answers to the following types of questions is important when screening for compulsive exercising:

- Do they exercise when sick or injured?
- Does it ruin their day if they cannot exercise?
- Do they miss social functions because they have to work out?
- Do they have to do a set routine or the workout does not count?
- Does walking count as exercise?

Compulsive exercisers seldom come in saying they have a problem with their level of activity. There are several reasons for this. They don't identify it as a problem, they don't want it tampered with, and if they are told to exercise less, they fear they will get fat. The fear of exercising less is terrifying to the compulsive exerciser.

THE TERMINOLOGY

Many terms are used to describe over-exercising.

> *Compulsive exercise, dysfunctional exercise, and activity disorder.* Individuals who continue to over-exercise in spite of medical and/or other consequences, or feel as if they cannot stop, are individuals who struggle with compulsive exercise. Dysfunctional exercise and activity disorder are two other terms used to describe compulsive exercise.[4]

> *Pathogenic exercise or exercise addiction.* These terms are used to describe individuals who are consumed by the need for physical activity to the exclusion of everything else and to the point of damage or danger to their lives.

> *Anorexia athletica.* This term is used to describe a sub-clinical eating disorder for athletes who engage in at least one unhealthy method of weight control, including fasting, vomiting, diet pills, laxatives, or diuretics.[5]

Primary exercise dependence. This term describes individuals who are addicted to exercise for reasons associated with doing the activity. For example, the compulsive runner whose running has become an end rather than means to an end, such as training for a marathon.

Secondary exercise dependence. This occurs when individuals use exercise to control and manipulate their body composition. They have an intense fear of becoming overweight and they exercise to burn calories. Another example of secondary exercise dependence is when the individuals want to increase the size of their physique and fear the loss of muscle. Secondary exercise dependence can co-occur with eating disorders and steroid use.[6]

BRAIN CHANGES

What effect does exercise have on the brain? Exercise is always touted as something healthy that everyone should do. When and why does that change? Serotonin, a neurotransmitter, is directly affected by food intake. Exercise, in addition to food intake, also affects serotonin levels; serotonin levels typically increase in the body as a result of exercising. This increase in levels is thought to have a reaction in the brain similar to the effects of taking antidepressants. Dopamine is another neurotransmitter affected by exercise. This is an excitatory neurotransmitter which gives us pleasure and reward. When we do something pleasurable such as exercise, we get a dopamine spike in the brain. Endorphins are neurotransmitters also affected by exercise, they are responsible for the euphoria also known as the "runner's high." They are powerful natural pain relievers which is why an individual can continue to exercise at a very high level without adequately fueling the body and not be exhausted or in pain. The combination of the "runner's high" (increased endorphin levels), feeling more pleasure and reward (elevated dopamine levels), and in a better mood (increased serotonin), makes compulsive exercising a very difficult behavior to break.

What Happens in the Eating Disordered Brain

In moderation, exercise can be a very useful tool to help an individual recover from addiction or eating disorder. As stated previously, physical activity has a beneficial effect on the brain's dopamine system, which is located in the reward center in the brain. The problem is that in the brain of the eating disordered individual, dopamine and serotonin may work differently. A person with both Anorexia Nervosa and Bulimia Nervosa experiences serotonin and dopamine malfunction in the areas of the brain that communicate hunger, pain, and taste to the body. They can also contribute to a distorted perception of the body. It is very common to have patients report that as soon as they eat something "fattening", they can actually see their thighs get bigger or "see" fat growing on their bodies. Research by Walter Kaye has shown that the magnitude of the serotonin and dopamine disturbance is greater in Anorexia Nervosa than in schizophrenia.[7]

How Exercise Affects the Eating Disordered Brain

Exercise increases the activity of neurotransmitter systems that are involved in the addictive process, including dopamine, serotonin, and endorphins. Because dopamine is the neurotransmitter associated with pleasure and reward, the development of the addiction occurs when the increased dopamine signals the pleasure part of the brain. As this pathway is reinforced through repeated drug exposures (compulsive exercise), the brain continues to initiate the behaviors (compulsive exercise) that led to the drug-induced neurotransmitter release.[8]

In other words, individuals who compulsively exercise increase the dopamine levels in their brains, signaling the desire to exercise more and more. The more individuals exercise, the more hard-wired or addicted to exercise they become. Initially, the increase in activity level is done with the intention of helping lose some weight or be a little healthier; the addiction appears to occur over time. Since the body is malnourished, its ability to increase serotonin and dopamine levels through its normal mechanism is compromised. It may be that the only way to increase the level of dopamine is through exercise.

CORTISOL: THE FEARED HORMONE

Cortisol is a hormone affected by stress and exercise. This hormone is identified as our chronic stress hormone; it contributes to cell death and remodeling of brain cells. When an individual is faced with chronic stress, the body has a high level of cortisol. This can be damaging to the brain and also leads to the body storing additional abdominal fat. Both emotional and physical stress (such as moderate or vigorous levels of exercise) can cause the brain to release more cortisol. The body adapts to this if it is fed; however, a starved or underfed body is also a stressed body. The combination of restricted intake and a moderate or vigorous level of exercise cause the body to produce more cortisol.[9] Long term elevation of cortisol levels causes a decrease in blood flow, oxygen, and glucose to the brain. This leads to a loss of neurons, shrinkage of the brain, and trouble concentrating.[10]

THE ROLE OF THE EATING DISORDER VOICE

Individuals who struggle with compulsive exercise are typically very competitive, driven, and self-disciplined. They operate with a "no pain, no gain" mentality. Days off are unheard of and they pride themselves in their ability to persevere. This plays right into the messages of the eating disorder voice: **"Whatever you do isn't good enough," "You can always do better," "You are weak," "You are lazy," "You're going to get fat."** These voices, combined with the addictive component of the exercise, help perpetuate the behavior. The drive to exercise almost always outweighs the logic.

Sarah's story is an example of how troubling the eating disorder voice can be for individuals who are compulsive exercisers.

Sarah's Story

Sarah, a 14-year-old patient, was diagnosed with Anorexia Nervosa. She had developed two stress fractures over the past six months, both of which were not healed. She had been put in a boot cast and told not to exercise. Her physician told her she wouldn't heal if she ran. In the evening after her parents went to bed, she would take her boot off and go for a five-mile run. Her parents eventually caught her. Much to their dismay, not only could they no longer trust her, but they also realized how much the disorder had taken over their daughter.

Sarah said it was easier to deal with getting into trouble than have to listen to the eating disorder voice. She described hearing, **"You're fat, lazy, and weak," "You can run and you have to run,"** and **"They are only telling you not to run so you can gain weight and get fat."** The only time she got relief was after she ran, and then she could fall asleep.

WARNING SIGNS OF COMPULSIVE EXERCISE
- Feeling anxious, guilty, and/or get angry if unable to exercise.
- Avoiding social functions interfering with exercise routine.
- Restricting food intake if not able to exercise, or exercising to compensate for food consumed.
- Exercising in addition to the training required for their sport.
- Counting only strenuous exercise, i.e. walking doesn't count.
- Exercising when sick or injured.
- No menstrual period for 3 or more months.
- Having one or more stress fractures without a significant injury.

BEYOND THE WARNING SIGNS
When individuals over-train or exercise daily to the point of exhaustion, their immune systems can be compromised by pouring the powerful stress hormones adrenaline and cortisol into their bodies. Exercising at a high level and not fueling the body adequately will lead to physical exhaustion. It has no time to rest and heal, and it increases the likelihood of injury, sickness and fatigue. Physiological and psychological complications are also associated with compulsive exercise.

Physiological Changes and Complications
When compulsive exercisers do not consume enough calories, they become catabolic—the body uses its own lean tissue as fuel. When not fed enough, the body will use lean tissue from different parts of the body including the

heart, bones, brain, and muscles in order to survive, resulting in one or more of the following:

Amenorrhea. Females who exercise compulsively may disrupt the balance of hormones in their bodies, which can change their menstrual cycles. When the percentage of body fat is too low, the body can't afford to spend calories on producing extra blood cells.

Osteopenia/osteoporosis. These occur when there is a thinning of the bones (which typically comes with normal aging). Female athletes who are amenorrheic are at high risk for bone loss.

Cardiac complications. Cardiac arrest is a potential consequence for someone who compulsively exercises and struggles with an eating disorder. The malnutrition and electrolyte imbalance put that individual at high risk for a cardiac event.

Neurological and Psychological Complications

Neurological and psychological changes and complications include the following:

Depression and anxiety. When individuals who struggle with compulsive exercise are unable to exercise, they suffer from an increased level of depression and anxiety.

Fatigue and insomnia. Individuals who compulsively exercise may also suffer from fatigue and insomnia.

Social isolation. As individuals become much more addicted to exercise, they begin to socially isolate themselves. They will avoid social functions if they interfere with their exercise routine. They put their need to exercise in front of anything else they need/want to do.

RELATIVE ENERGY DEFICIT IN SPORTS (RED-S)

A person, male or female, who plays sports or exercise intensely may be at risk for Relative Energy Deficit in Sports (RED-S). Relative Energy Deficit in Sports refers to impaired physiological function including, but not limited to, metabolic rate, menstrual function, bone health, immunity, protein synthesis, cardiovascular health caused by relative energy deficit.

Since the primary cause of Relative Energy Deficit in Sports is under-fueling, the condition is most common in cross-country running, gymnastics, ballet, figure skating, and sports that have weight classes, such as rowing.11 (foot note) These athletes may not realize how many calories they burn during workouts and don't eat enough to maintain a positive energy balance. Someone may try, as well as be encouraged to by coaches, parents, and team-mates, to lose weight in order to look and/or perform better. They may skip meals or avoid fatty foods or specific food groups, causing an energy deficit resulting in muscle loss, fatigue, and poor performance.

Exercising intensely and not eating enough calories can lead to a decrease in estrogen, the hormone that helps to regulate the menstrual cycle. As a result, a girl's periods may become irregular or stop altogether.[12, 13] Female athletes often welcome the absence of regular periods, but this is not normal, acceptable, nor desirable. When periods stop, the body is communicating that something is wrong. Normal monthly periods should be the goal for all female athletes—in all sports and at all levels of competition.

Osteoporosis is a weakening of the bones due to the loss of bone density and improper bone formation. Low estrogen levels, poor nutrition, especially low calcium intake, and low vitamin D levels can lead to osteoporosis. This condition can ruin an athlete's career because it may lead to stress fractures and other injuries.[14]

If someone who is diagnosed with Relative Energy Deficit in Sports is informed and able to eat enough to correct the metabolic rate, gets within normal ranges of the BCA, and if female has regular periods, that person is not a compulsive exerciser. A compulsive exerciser has an addiction that is harder to treat and often has several physiological functions reduced.

THE USEFULNESS OF METABOLIC TESTING
AND BODY COMPOSITION ANALYSIS

Maria's story below highlights how Metabolic Testing and Body Composition Analysis are used in diagnosing and developing a treatment plan for a compulsive exerciser. It shows the effectiveness of seeing the tests results in motivating the patient to follow our recommendations.

Maria's Story

Maria, a 17-year-old girl, was five feet tall and weighed 95 pounds. She was on the varsity crew team and practiced two hours every day for the nationals. She had her first period when she was 14; over the last three years she had a total of 10 periods. She was eating 1,400 calories a day and wanted to weigh 90 pounds. She weighed herself at least twice a day. If the scale was up one day, she made sure it was down the following day. Two years earlier, she had a stress fracture, but no bone density test had been done. Metabolic Testing showed she was severely hypo-metabolic, burning only 386 calories a day and therefore using her own lean tissue (organs, muscle, and bone) for fuel. Other medical tests revealed that she was anemic, deficient in vitamin D, and had osteopenia (bone loss).

Initially, she reluctantly agreed to eat 2,000 calories a day. She was asked to stop exercising in order to correct the Relative Energy Deficit in Sports. After two months she got her period, and after four months of eating close to 2,200 calories a day, she had reached 100 pounds. This scared her. Her Metabolic Test and Body Composition Analysis showed major improvements, but her metabolism was still not corrected. She felt that she should be rewarded, and her parents allowed and encouraged her to start exercising again. Three weeks later she was re-tested and her metabolic rate had plummeted down from 1,100 calories to 437 calories a day. She had lost lean mass and her fat weight had increased. She had returned to being very hypometabolic and catabolic. It's as if her body was saying: **"Don't mess with me... I'll show you, you are hurting yourself!"**

Maria and her parents were wrong in thinking that just because she had reached 100 pounds and had gotten her period that she was recovered. It took another three months, eating 2,500 calories per day, for her body to recover and to have a normal metabolic rate with a healthy amount of lean mass. She ended up weighing just over 100 pounds. Her percentage of body fat was lower than at her first visit. She admitted that she had been in denial and would have continued being in denial if it wasn't for the Metabolic Testing and the Body Composition Analysis.

This case study illustrates how compulsive exercisers who do not consume enough calories become catabolic. In our practices, we use Metabolic Testing and Body Composition Analysis to respectively measure how the body has been affected by a high level of exercise and inadequate nutritional intake. The Body Composition Analysis helps us assess what effect the behaviors have had on the skeleton and muscle. Although we are not able to measure how much muscle or bone has been lost as a result of over-exercise, we are able to see if their fat-free mass, including bone and muscle, is below the minimum level.

The combination of these tests is extremely helpful in convincing individuals they are doing harm to their bodies. It is difficult to convince compulsive exercisers that their excessive exercise may be damaging to their body. When they are faced with the data that shows their bodies being hypometabolic and catabolic, despite working out for more than two hours a day, they are more likely to follow the treatment recommendations. The ongoing test results help convince them that cutting back on exercise and eating more lead to increased energy and improved health. Without the test results, patients often indicate they would not have entertained making any of the changes.

Questions and Answers for Compulsive Exercise

Q: Is there such a thing as too much exercise?

A: Yes, federal guidelines recommend 20 to 45 minutes of aerobic activity five to six days a week, burning 2,000 to 3,500 calories per week. Exercising more than one hour a day over five days per week is considered extreme for most people. There will be times when you will go for a three- or four-hour hike, but it is the consistent daily level that can be excessive. Athletes will exercise five to six days a week for two hours or more. This is not considered excessive if they are eating enough.

Q: Why are females who exercise prone to bone loss when exercise is recommended to increase bone density?

A: Osteoporosis is a weakening of the bones due to the loss of bone density or improper bone formation. Low estrogen levels, poor nutrition (especially low calcium intake), and low vitamin D levels can lead to osteoporosis. An athlete's bone health reflects her cumulative history of calories consumed and menstrual status, as well as her genetics. Girls gain more than 50 percent of skeletal mass during adolescence and reach peak bone mass between 18 and 25 years of age. Bones weaken as the number of missed menstrual cycles accumulates, and this loss may not be fully reversible. The risk for stress fracture is two to four times greater in amenorrheic athletes compared to those who regularly menstruate.[14]

Q: Are males also at risk for bone loss?

A: Yes, males are also at risk, but females are at a higher risk. If calcium intake is low and calorie intake is not adequate for the activity level, any individual is at risk for not having proper bone formation or bone loss.

Q: Does the metabolic rate change with increased exercise?

A: It depends on how much the individual eats. If the exercise is at a high level and the food intake covers the extra expense, then the body will be hypermetabolic. If the body is underfed, it may be hypometabolic. The point is that the body does not necessarily burn more calories with increased activity unless it is fed properly.

Q: What type of exercise "doesn't count"?

A: Individuals who struggle with compulsive exercise will not count any activity that will not make them sweat or give them an "endorphin kick." All types of exercise count; i.e., daily walking, gardening, etc.

CHAPTER 8

Other Specified Feeding and
Eating Disorders (OSFED)

"I have severely restricted my intake for years, always less than 1,000 calories, but often less than 600 calories a day. Despite how little I eat, I never get to a low weight. I drive myself crazy, counting the calories, obsessing about what I can and can't eat, and weighing myself five to 10 times a day."

– Debbie, diagnosed with Atypical AN

"I don't think I really have a problem; I only make myself throw up if I eat too much. It only happens two or three times a month. That's how I keep from gaining weight."

– Sue, diagnosed with Sub-Threshold BN

"I am really good about following my diet plan, but every two to three weeks I just have to eat everything in sight. Afterward, I usually don't eat the next day and then am back on my diet plan."

– Jody, diagnosed with Sub-Threshold BED

"I know I don't binge, but I have to make myself throw up when my stomach feels full. If I get stressed out, I can't relax until I have thrown up. When my stomach feels empty, I can concentrate. It helps me control my anxiety."

– Lori, diagnosed with Purging Disorder

"I'm waking up in the middle of the night and some-times not even aware of the quantity I ate until the next morning. It's only because I find the dirty dishes and the food wrappers that I know how much I consumed."

– Carol, diagnosed with Night Eating Syndrome

OSFED SUB-TYPES

The above testimonials from our patients show a range of behaviors that often leave individuals who engage in them confused, distressed, and unsure as to why it's happening to them. They are all involved in a sub-type of an eating disorder that is included in the DSM-5 as Other Specified Eating and Feeding Disorders (OSFED). These sub-types include Atypical Anorexia Nervosa, Sub-Threshold Bulimia Nervosa, Sub-Threshold Binge Eating Disorder, Purging Disorder, and Night Eating Disorder. Even though these disorders may appear to be less severe because they do not meet the full criteria for Anorexia Nervosa, Bulimia Nervosa, or Binge Eating Disorder, they are at high risk for medical complications and are often overlooked.

According to the DSM-5 criteria, to be diagnosed as having OSFED, a person must present with a feeding or eating behavior that causes clinically significant distress and impairment in the areas of functioning, but does not meet the full criteria for any of the other feeding and eating disorders. While this criterion provides a better path for clinicians to properly diagnose symptoms, it is still very difficult for these patients to initially present for treatment and discuss what they are struggling with.

OSFED is one of the categories in the DSM-5 that will hopefully promote earlier diagnosis and treatment. Previously, the category "Eating Disorders, Not Otherwise Specified (EDNOS)", a diagnostic group in the

DSM-IV, often left patients feeling that they were "not that sick." Insurance companies or third- party payers are partly to blame for this, because it was more difficult for patients in this category to get insurance coverage for treatment of their illness.

Unfortunately, individuals who fit into the OSFED diagnostic group often hesitate to seek treatment. They feel they have failed at trying to lose weight because of their unhealthy eating habits. Their blood work is often normal and their body weight is not critically low, so they are often over-looked or misdiagnosed. They hesitate to bring up their problem to their medical provider because they do not look sick. However, simply because the body weight might not be critically low or the frequency of binging and purging is not more than once a week, they are still at high risk for medical complications and are often not diagnosed. A study done by Crow, and colleagues (2009) found that mortality in the EDNOS patient popula-tion (which includes OSFED) was actually higher in this group than in Anorexia Nervosa or Bulimia Nervosa.[1]

OSFED DISORDERS

The following eating disorders are included in the OSFED diagnostic group. The criteria for each as outlined in the DSM-5 are as follows:[2]

> *Atypical Anorexia Nervosa.* The individual meets criteria for Anorexia Nervosa, except that body weight is not substantially lower than normal or expected. An indi-vidual may be normal- or above-normal body weight in spite of having severely restricted their intake for several years.

> *Sub-Threshold Bulimia Nervosa (of low frequency and/ or limited duration).* This individual meets criteria for Bulimia Nervosa, except that the binge eating and com-pensatory behaviors have taken place for fewer than three months, or occur less than once per week.

> *Sub-Threshold Binge Eating Disorder (of low frequency and/or limited duration).* This individual meets criteria for

Binge Eating Disorder, except that the binge eating has taken place for fewer than three months, or occurs less than once per week.

Purging Disorder. This individual exhibits regular purging (e.g., vomiting, laxatives, and/or diuretics) at least once a week for at least three months, but in the absence of binge eating.

Night Eating Syndrome. This individual exhibits repeated episodes of night eating, such as waking up in the middle of the night to eat, or consuming an excessive amount of calories after the evening meal.

Atypical Anorexia Nervosa

Sara's story is a good example of how someone with Atypical Anorexia Nervosa benefited from Metabolic Testing.

Sara's Story

Sara is a 30-year-old female who restricted her intake for many years; at 5'8" she weighed 240 pounds. She initially came for an evaluation in hopes of seeing why she could not lose weight. She typically skipped breakfast, ate a sandwich and yogurt for lunch, and had a low-calorie frozen meal and fruit for dinner—totaling less than 1,200 calories per day. She was always being encouraged by her physician to lose weight, and would often hear the lecture regarding the health risks of being overweight. Metabolic Testing showed she was hypometabolic, burning only 925 calories per day, and catabolic, with a protein turnover of 38 percent, normal being 15 percent.

She was intensely fearful of gaining weight and avoided going out in public because of how much she despised how she looked. She was diagnosed with Atypical Anorexia Nervosa.

The Metabolic Testing and Body Composition Analysis were helpful in allowing her to identify that she had been under-eating. She always thought if she ate more than 1,200 calories, she was overeating and would gain more weight. Sara was skeptical about increasing her intake but did finally agree to eat more, initially increasing her intake to 2,000 calories a day. When she saw she didn't gain weight, but actually improved in lean weight and decreased her fat weight, she began to trust her body. She noticed improvements in her energy and began to exercise more regularly.

Eventually, she was able to increase her intake to 2,400 calories per day. Her metabolic rate took approximately ten weeks to correct. In the process, she lost 10 pounds of body fat and improved her lean weight.

CHALLENGES WITH TREATING OSFED PATIENTS

As nutritionists, our experience is that patients with OSFED respond very well to treatment—the real challenge is early diagnosis and intervention. It is difficult to identify this patient population and convince them they need treatment. Whenever we do an educational program, at the end of the presentation individuals come forth and say, **"I never knew I had a problem, but you just described me,"** or **"I've struggled with this all my life, but no one ever thought it was a problem."** If individuals are normal body weight or overweight, the focus is now on a healthy BMI (Body Mass Index) in their annual physical. This discourages patients from talking about what they struggle with; they just see their behaviors as a means to an end, saying, **"It's how I regulate my weight. If I didn't do this [purge after a big meal], I'd gain weight."** As health-care providers we need to recognize that any individual can be at risk to develop an eating disorder.

So many of the behaviors OFSED patients use almost become a normal routine for them, **"If I occasionally overeat, I just throw it up so I don't gain weight."** These behaviors are very secretive and family members are seldom aware of the struggles. What family or support individuals do notice is how negative or critical individuals with OFSED are about their looks and/or weight. They are always commenting on wanting to lose weight, feeling guilty about eating certain foods, and frequently dieting; they feel very ashamed about not being able to lose weight.

Patients often come in for weight loss help and are diagnosed with OSFED. It is a relief for them to finally know that they struggle with a disease—it's not about "willpower." **"I just thought I didn't have the willpower to follow a diet."** It's not unusual that they are initially very successful dieters, but always regain the weight lost because it is about much more than the food.

In the case study of Sara, she had always been counseled about how to lose weight. When she was assessed and told she had been under-eating, she was relieved; previous recommendations had always been about how to eat healthier and what she needed to do to lose weight. She expressed finally feeling like she was being heard and was able to receive the help she needed.

Individuals who fall into the DSM-5 category of OSFED are difficult for the clinician to recognize. Unless questions are asked specifically about their relationship between food and their bodies, they will not be identified. This patient population seldom recognizes that their behavior is unhealthy and not normal. They do not feel they are seen and do not believe they deserve treatment. Their belief is, **"I'm not that sick."** Their obsessive thoughts about body image, food, and exercise are typically very strong (their eating disorder voice) and this is why they turn to these behaviors.

By the time individuals come in for help, their body's response to the treatment recommendations can be compromised. Individuals who have weight-cycled or yo-yo dieted for years may have difficulty achieving a lower body weight. Their body's natural set point has probably increased over the years because of the weight cycling. However, they can develop a much healthier relationship to food and no longer weight cycle. These are individuals who have starved their body for years in a variety of ways that did not result in a significant drop in body weight.. Because of the normal or above-normal body weight, no one realized they had an eating problem.

Physiological Changes And Complications

Individuals who are diagnosed with OSFED suffer physiological changes very similar to those who suffer from Anorexia Nervosa, Bulimia Nervosa, or Binge Eating Disorder. Although their behaviors are not frequent or severe enough to classify them in these categories, the effect on the body can be just as severe.

> *Gastrointestinal complaints.* These may include gastric reflux, feeling full, bloating, constipation, diarrhea, and/or esophagitis.

> *Cardiac complications.* Cardiac complications may include a low potassium level, which can cause heart irregularity.

> *Other complications.* Other complications that might arise are associated with obesity and weight gain, such as high cholesterol levels, Type 2 diabetes, hypertension, and heart disease.

Neurological and Psychological Changes and Complications

Individuals who are diagnosed with OSFED may suffer from depression, anxiety, and obsessive-compulsive traits. They may also experience poor memory and concentration.

THE USEFULNESS OF METABOLIC TESTING
AND BODY COMPOSITION ANALYSIS

> *"The initial reason I went in for help was that no matter how increasingly little I ate, I was gaining weight. Looking back, I see it was extremely hard to stay at such a low weight. I had been eating less than 1,200 calories a day and the weight was still creeping up. The testing was very helpful and a rock-solid way of measuring progress. That*

helped me see the correlation between food and health, not just food and weight. I used to weigh myself at least two times a day, now I have no idea how much I weigh. My increased energy and uplifted mood are extremely helpful in motivating me. Yes, it's been difficult gaining and not knowing when the end was going to be. I eventually started to think, what does it matter if I go up a size or two if I feel this strong and healthy and my metabolism is normal; it's all worth it!"

– Louise

Metabolic Testing and Body Composition Analysis are extremely helpful when working with these patients. This is a group who look normal and no one would suspect that they were malnourished or had an eating disorder. However, the majority of these individuals are hypometabolic and catabolic. Their body has slowed down because it is being under-fed and is using its own protein stores to fuel itself. Many of these individuals are normal body weight or above normal body weight and have been trying to regulate their weight by restricting their intake or purging if they overeat. They believe that they need to eat fewer calories to maintain or lose weight. The Metabolic Testing provides "proof" that they need to increase their intake.

The BCA is especially useful because initially it can guide us in our treatment recommendations. Individuals diagnosed with OSFED who have typically been trying to follow a 1,200-calorie diet have been under-fed long-term and are often malnourished. With those individuals, the BCA allows us to see how much fat-free mass they have. Based on this, we can make protein intake recommendations to help correct the malnourished state.

We use the BCA to guide us in our intake recommendations. Because of the starvation mode the body has been in, it may store fat very easily. Following the BCA on a weekly basis helps us guide our patients to restore their metabolic rate and minimize their fat weight gain. Without these two tests, it would be difficult to treat the OSFED patient population. Nutritionists and physicians often believe that individuals who are overweight tend to underestimate the size portions they consume and do not count all the food that they eat. This testing shows that they often are under-eating and need to increase their intake to burn more calories.

Working with this patient population has been very rewarding. By following their individualized meal plan, based on their BCA, they experience a significant decrease in their symptoms. Similar to the patient testimonial below, our OSFED patients often feel relieved that they are no longer using unhealthy eating behaviors and start to feel better about themselves.

"I came to the clinic after a lifetime of being on a weight gain-loss roller coaster. For the first time in my life, I even considered bariatric surgery, but was concerned that my self-esteem would suffer if I took that "easy way out." I had lost weight on 30 or more plans previously, some with radical fasting programs, so I knew I could lose the needed weight. But in the past, I gained back everything I had lost—plus a good deal more. I had to learn to eat in a very different way. I usually skipped breakfast to "save" calories for later in the day. Now I was front-loading the day and feeling much better throughout the day. My progress has been slow but steady. I have the occasional over-indulgent weeks, but it's not a huge setback because I know that my new lifestyle is both manageable and effective."

– Lois

Questions and Answers for OSFED

Q: Why do all the magazines indicate that a healthy diet for someone who wants to lose weight is 1,200 calories?

A: Many things mentioned in magazines are not accurate. Each individual needs to have a plan based on his or her body's needs. Several factors need to be considered, including height, body weight, fat-free mass, medical problems, and activity level. Diets are not a one-size-fits-all. The body needs a minimum of 1200 calories daily for organs to function properly in the resting state, majority of adults need well above that.

Q: Why do I gain weight on more than 1,200 calories?

A: You will gain weight if you are hypometabolic and consume more calories than you burn. The metabolic rate needs to be corrected in order not to continue to gain weight. If you front-load the day and increase your protein intake, your metabolic rate will take less time to correct.

Q: If I eat, will I just keep gaining weight?

A: If you are hypometabolic and you increase your intake, you may have some initial weight gain. However, as your metabolic rate increases, you will gradually begin to lose fat weight.

Q: Why do I eat in the middle of the night, sometimes without even being aware?

A: If you struggle with nighttime eating or binging, it may be an indication that your intake is not adequate during the day. It is important to front-load your day and eat the recommended amount of calories. Working with an eating disorder treatment team can assist you to understand and treat this problem.

Q: I have Type 2 diabetes and my doctor wants me to lose weight. Regardless of how little I eat, I can't lose weight. What can I do?

A: Type 2 diabetes makes it much more difficult to lose weight. Severely restricting your intake will only make it more difficult to lose weight long-term. You may initially lose some weight, but the majority will be lean tissue. When you increase your calorie intake, you will gain fat weight. It is important to work with a dietitian/nutritionist to determine your metabolic needs and develop an eating and exercise plan to achieve healthy weight loss.

Q: Is there a healthy way to lose weight?

A: There can be, but the body has regulatory mechanisms to resist weight loss. Many diets claim they are a healthy approach to losing weight, however, the majority of the weight lost is typically lean weight or muscle. When this occurs, the body is very quick to respond by becoming hypometabolic. All weight lost is usually regained as well as extra pounds within a short period of time. The body is designed to survive, so severely restricting its food intake (necessary for survival) sets off mechanisms in the body to resist long-term weight loss and actually increase overall body fat. It is important to understand what is a healthy weight for your body. Trying to lose a few pounds for cosmetic reasons may result in long term weight cycling.

CHAPTER 9

Healthy Eating

"I've always eaten healthily—lots of fresh fruits, veg-etables, and lean proteins, rarely any soda, candy, condi-ments, or creamy sauces—so nutritionists basically said, "Keep doing what you're doing." It was only when I met Annika that I realized how wrong they were! Yes, I ate healthy things, but no, I was not a healthy eater!"

– Paige

NUTRITION: THE CORNERSTONE OF OUR PRACTICES

Throughout this book we have reminded readers that we are nutritionists; we see nutrition, proper nutritional assessment, and healthy eating as an integral part of our treatment protocol when working with eating disor-dered individuals. The key to healthy eating is getting the right amount of calories and nutrients to sustain a healthy body. However, the patient popu-lations we work with are often suffering from malnutrition when they first come through our doors. Many of them have either starved their bodies, have become under-nourished because of an inadequate food intake, have purged to the point of being semi-starved, and/or have compulsively exercised and have not eaten enough calories, causing them to become malnourished. Others, like the woman who wrote the testimonial above, are not necessarily misusing food, but their definition of "healthy eating" has led them to being almost malnourished. As we have stated throughout this book, when the body is not properly nourished, it is susceptible to becoming hypometabolic and/or catabolic, which are both indicators of malnutrition.

Part of our high success rate in treating patients can be attributed to extracting the nutritional information we need from Metabolic Testing and Body Composition Analysis in order to see first-hand whether or not they suffer from malnutrition. It is the starting point. Healthy eating not only sustains the body but also creates an environment where the body can begin to heal both emotionally and physically. This is critical for optimum brain function. Neurotransmitter levels are dependent on a healthy intake as these levels decrease when the body is malnourished. In order for the brain to heal, the body needs proper nutrition. Because healthy eating is such a critical component for the well-being of our patients, it has become the cornerstone of our practices.

WHAT THE BODY NEEDS TO FUNCTION

We need food for three main reasons:

1. For energy, which our body requires to power all activity.
2. To promote growth and repair of bodily tissues.
3. To regulate vital processes within the body.

To function properly and meet its nutritional needs, the body needs an adequate amount of macronutrients, including protein, carbohydrates, and fat. It also needs the right fuel (food) and regular maintenance (exercise and healthy lifestyle) to operate at optimum level. How individuals eat affects their immune system, delays the effects of aging, enhances their ability to concentrate and focus, affects their mood, wards off serious illnesses, promotes the body's healing ability, and gives them the energy and vitality they need to face life's challenges.

A BALANCED FOOD PLAN

The role of the nutritionist is to put together a balanced food plan for optimal health. This is one of the key components of our treatment plans when working with patients who have eating disorders. Since our philosophy is to measure health from within, we design individualized food plans for each and every patient with the intention to make sure their bodies are receiving the nutrition needed for optimal health. All food plans must have a balanced proportion of protein, fats, and carbohydrates, which will be discussed below.

Protein

For decades it has been said that a calorie is just a calorie, but when re-feeding a malnourished body the right quality and quantity of calories or foods are needed to rebuild healthy cell mass. Protein is of primary importance: 0.7 to 0.8 grams of protein per pound of body weight, spread out evenly throughout the day, is crucial. The requisite amount is based on weight and body composition. Those who weigh more or have more muscle have more tissue to maintain and thus will have higher protein needs. Protein is intricately involved in every part and function of the body. It is needed for growth and maintenance of muscles, brain, immune system, blood, intestines, enzymes, bone, skin, hair, nails, teeth, hormones, and organ cells.[1]

The quality of protein is important in building the body's lean tissue. Nine essential amino acids, the building blocks of protein, must come from food; the body naturally makes the other 13 amino acids for a total of 22 needed for protein synthesis (building lean tissue). If only one essential amino acid is missing, protein cannot be built. Animal and soy proteins provide all the nine essential amino acids (referred to as "complete protein"), but the amino acids in starches, nuts, legumes, and vegetables are incomplete. To build lean tissue without animal foods, the foods must balance each other to provide all nine essential amino acids.[2] This is why vegetarian diets take more planning and effort. Some vegetarian combinations that provide all nine essential amino acids are; dairy + grains, grains + legumes, legumes + seeds, and grains + deep-colored vegetables.[3]

Fat

Eating fat does not make you fat. In fact, fat is essential for good nutrition, just as vitamins are. Unfortunately, years of anti-fat messages from health authorities concerned about the supposed link between dietary fat and heart disease have led a lot of people today to think it is healthier to eliminate fat. We have created a fat-phobic society. A growing number of people, including many of our patients, eat too little fat to maintain healthy body functions, such as vitamin absorption, hormone production, and normal brain function.

Individuals with eating disorders often take the anti-fat message too far. They believe that if low-fat eating is good, then no-fat eating must be even better. A common barrier to change is their belief that dietary fat has no nutritional value and is automatically converted to body fat. They are also aware that a gram of fat has 9 calories, while a gram of protein or carbohydrates has only 4 calories. They feel that by sharply reducing the amount of fat in their diet, they are avoiding unnecessary calories and weight gain. However, fat is essential in the diet and can also prevent common diseases, like cancer, heart disease, and stroke.[4,5,6] A healthy diet should include at least 30 percent of the total calories from fat. In a 2,000-calorie diet, for example, there should be at least 60 to 65 grams of fat.

Patients are often surprised to learn that they can develop a dietary deficiency by avoiding fat. We depend on fat to get essential fatty acids and if we do not get enough on a daily basis, deficiencies often occur. Symptoms include dry, cracked, and scaling skin; brittle nails; hair loss and dull hair; being cold; impaired wound healing; loss of menses or increased premenstrual symptoms; and constipation and/or diarrhea.[7] Having adequate fat intake is also very important for cognitive function, concentration, and stable moods.

Carbohydrates

The major function of carbohydrates is to provide a continuous energy supply to the trillions of cells within the body. Carbohydrates are the main source of blood glucose, which is a major fuel for all of the body's cells and the only source of energy for the brain and red blood cells. Glucose is essential for the proper functioning of the nervous system. The symptoms of lowered blood glucose, or hypoglycemia, include feelings of weakness, hunger, and dizziness.

Forty to 60 percent of total daily calories should come from carbohydrates. In a 2,000-calorie diet, for example, there should be 200 to 300 grams of carbohydrates.[8]

Carbohydrates are divided into simple and complex carbohydrates. Simple carbohydrates, sometimes called simple sugars, include fructose (fruit sugar), sucrose (table sugar), and lactose (milk sugar), as well as several other sugars. Fruits are one of the richest natural sources of simple carbohydrates. Complex carbohydrates are also made up of sugars, but the sugar molecules are strung together to form longer, more complex chains. Complex carbohydrates include fiber and starches. Foods rich in complex carbohydrates include vegetables, whole grains, peas, and beans. Except for fiber, which cannot be digested, both simple and complex carbohydrates are converted into glucose. Glucose is then either used directly to provide energy for the body, or it is stored in the liver for further use.

Fiber

Fiber falls into two types: soluble and insoluble. Soluble fiber is found in oat bran, barley, nuts, seeds, beans, lentils, peas and some fruit and vegetables. It attracts water and turns to gel during digestion, and is commonly found in fiber supplements. Insoluble fiber is found in wheat bran, vegetables, and whole grains and does not dissolve in water. It adds bulk to the stool and helps food pass more quickly through the stomach and intestines.[9] The combination of soluble and insoluble fiber is important in keeping the gastrointestinal tract functioning. Some individuals struggling with an eating disorder consume large amounts of fiber. Fiber slows down digestion, which results in feeling full much longer.

We have seen that extremely high fiber intake causes the metabolic rate to decrease significantly, which also interferes with the absorption of valuable nutrients. The 2005 Dietary Guidelines for Americans recommend approximately 25 grams fiber daily.

THE USEFULNESS OF METABOLIC TESTING
AND BODY COMPOSITION ANALYSIS

Some of our patients are in denial of how under-nourished they actually are, either when we first meet them or through the recovery process. Metabolic Testing and Body Composition Analysis serve as a wake-up call or a reality check for many of them to truly understand what is going on with the nutritional status of their body. In addition to eating disorder patients, we assess all the patients we treat. Many of them have been found to be malnourished due to under-eating. Regardless of whether the under-eating was intentional or not, the effect on the body has been the same. Without those two tests, those patients would not have been effectively treated. Identifying an individual whose resting metabolic rate (RMR) is well below the predicted level helps us recognize that the individual is fueling the body inadequately. The combination of these two tests helps us not only with assessment, but also in providing the data needed to design individualized eating plans for each patient's, unique nutritional needs.

> *"My Metabolic Test showed I was hypometabolic, which meant my metabolic rate was lower than that of an average person, and the Body Composition Analysis showed that my fat mass was relatively high. This was alarming because I was a thin girl and always assumed I had a fast metabolism and low body fat. I would never have known that my body was stressed because I wasn't consuming enough calories."*
>
> *- Paige*

The Metabolic Test measures the individual's RMR, which varies depending on sex, height, weight, intake, and exercise level. Most healthy people will fall in the range of 1,200 to 2,000 calories a day. Additional calories are needed for physical activities.

Calories Needed to Maintain Healthy Organs and Tissues in Adults[10]

- Liver: ~ 485 kcal/day
- Brain: ~ 340 kcal/day
- Heart: ~ 125 kcal/day
- Kidneys: ~ 185 kcal/day
- Muscle: ~ 325 kcal/day

CORRECTING THE METABOLIC RATE
THROUGH BALANCED EATING

When correcting a metabolism that has slowed down (hypometabolic), we initially recommend increasing intake to a minimum of 1,500 to 2,000 calories per day. Anything less causes the metabolism to drop even further and the person may become catabolic (using lean mass for fuel/energy). As treatment continues, calories are increased depending on the body's response. It is not unusual to need 3,000 to 4,000 calories daily to repair the body. Even individuals who are at a healthy weight need to repair the physiological damage done to the body by the eating disorder behaviors.

Patients will often say, "I just want to eat when I'm hungry; isn't that the healthy way to eat?" For someone with a normal metabolic rate the answer is, "Yes, intuitive eating is healthy." However, a hypometabolic body will not be hungry in a healthy way. Such a person will have distorted hunger, will feel full much sooner, and will likely have gastric discomfort (stomach pain).

When individuals are hypometabolic, their digestion slows down and many suffer from gastroparesis (slow-moving gut).[11] Using digestive enzymes helps to break down the food. If an individual is eating less, then there will be less enzyme production, which results in food being digested much slower.[12] We have found that multi-enzyme formula and/or gastric digestive enzymes help alleviate some of the bloating that may occur. Discomfort decreases as the body is nourished, but normal and healthy hunger cues can often take a long time to return. To ultimately correct the metabolic rate, patients need to eat often, even when they are not hungry or when they feel full.

THE IMPORTANCE OF BREAKFAST AND
FRONT-LOADING CALORIES

Breakfast is the most important meal of the day. It is particularly important in correcting the metabolic rate, since skipping breakfast may slow down the metabolism. Patients often complain that eating breakfast makes them hungrier throughout the day. This may be true, because by eating more, the metabolic rate increases and they burn more calories throughout the day.

Ideally, one-third of the daily calorie and protein intake should be eaten by 11 a.m. and two-thirds by 3 to 4 p.m.

Front-loading the day with higher calories early on helps speed up the metabolism.[13] We have also found that it helps to decrease mouth hunger. Mouth hunger isn't true hunger; rather, it is a craving. This usually occurs later in the day and is caused by under-eating, especially protein, earlier in the day.

THE NEED TO CONSUME MORE CALORIES

As the metabolic rate increases and improves, the patient needs to consume more calories. This is often difficult and frightening for the individual with an eating disorder. The common fear is: **"If I eat more I will gain weight,"** or **"If I start eating I won't be able to stop."** The body's natural drive to restore weight and health often leads to what might feel like over-eating or binging for the individual. Consuming enough calories from a variety of foods creates more satiety and less desire to binge. When intake is restrictive, patients often experience a desire to overeat or binge despite feeling full.

The same is true for when the body is repairing damaged cells. Extra calories are needed, resulting in periods of increased or extreme hunger that might, once again be interpreted by a patient as causing bingeing. This is not a binge, but rather the body's way of saying that it needs more calories to heal and to restore health. Working with a nutritionist will help minimize these episodes. It is important to accept and respect that the body needs extra calories to restore the lean and fat stores, and that this is necessary for survival.

CHANGING ENERGY LEVELS

Patients experience an increase in fatigue when they first start to eat more. During this time, we encourage them to give the body the rest that it needs. Energy then begins to increase within a few weeks of improved eating. We often hear patients comment that they thought they would feel better when they started to eat more, but recovery requires patience. The body has experienced a significant amount of damage and needs to rest in order to heal. As intake increases and the metabolic rate improves, there will eventually be a significant increase in energy. Some patients describe the energy change as quite sudden. If no change in energy is experienced, it may indicate that the body is still hypometabolic.

SIGNS THE BODY IS REPAIRING ITSELF

> "It took several weeks, maybe even months, before I saw the results that I wanted. It took a lot of patience and trust. In the first few weeks my weight increased and my weekly body composition tests showed my fat and fat-free masses were both increasing. This was daunting because I thought that a change in my eating habits would cause my fat-free mass to increase and my fat mass to decrease. Annika continued to reassure me that everything was going according to plan. Eventually, my metabolic rate normalized and my body composition improved.
>
> – Paige

In our experience, it takes a minimum of six to eight weeks of healthy eating to correct the metabolic rate. For some patients, however, it can take much longer because of their malnourished state or the inability to consume needed calories. The body needs to repair at the cellular level and this takes time. The crucial markers that need to be tracked and monitored are metabolic rate measured by Metabolic Testing and cellular integrity and change in body lean mass measured by Body Composition Analysis.

We also see other physical changes that indicate that the body is improving. The basal body temperature will gradually increase and there will be less cold intolerance. Circulation in the hands and feet will improve and they will no longer be cool to the touch. The resting heart rate will increase, blood pressure will stabilize, and stomach and bowel function will improve. Medication or increased exercise cannot correct a malnourished or hypometabolic state; the only remedy is proper eating. A patient may have a lot of anxiety about increasing calories and that anxiety may be treated with medication, but nothing other than food will repair the body's nutritional status.

Questions and Answers for Healthy Eating

Q: How much protein do I need?

A: Most people will fall into the normal range for protein recommendation: 70 to 110 grams per day for women and 120 to 160 grams for men. Your individual recommendation depends on your amount of fat-free mass (test result from the Body Composition Analysis). The body will not use more than 40 to 45 grams at any given time, so it's important to spread it out throughout the day.

Q: Is there such a thing as eating too much fiber?

A: Yes. You might experience cramping, bloating, gas, and abdominal discomfort as your body attempts to work through the bulk. If you're not drinking enough water to help move the bulk through your system, constipation is common. If the constipation is not resolved it can lead to an intestinal blockage—the most dangerous side effect. Also, if you are eating too much fiber and neglecting other nutrients in the process, you may develop nutritional deficiencies over time. Many foods that are high in fiber typically contain plenty of carbohydrates but not much fat or protein. To avoid an imbalance, also eat protein-rich foods and healthy fats at each major meal and follow the recommendation of eating approximately 25 grams of fiber daily.

Q: If I am gluten intolerant or have celiac disease, what do I need to do differently?

A: Gluten is found in grains such as wheat, barley, and rye. A gluten-free diet is used to treat celiac disease. Gluten causes inflammation in the small intestines in people with celiac disease. Our advice is to work with a nutritionist and follow a gluten-free diet that helps control the signs and symptoms and prevents complications.

Q: I have PCOS. What should I do?

A: PCOS (polycystic ovary syndrome) is a metabolic disorder. Exactly why and how PCOS develops is not quite clear; however, the discovery of insulin's role has brought hopes for better treatment. If insulin resistance is present, it is best treated with diet and exercise, based on guidance from a nutritionist. Insulin- sensitizing medications may be used as well.

Q: If I take a multivitamin, does that meet my nutritional needs?

A: A multivitamin does not take the place of food. Vitamins and minerals in their natural form (food) are often more available to the body and absorbed much better. A multivitamin is not meant to be the sole source of nutrients.

Q: What signs should I look for to identify if I am malnourished?

A: Malnutrition is very difficult to identify. The body is designed to take care of nutritional deficiencies and often pulls from vital protein stores in the body to make sure that blood levels stay within a normal range. That is why blood work is often normal in the malnourished individual. Hair loss is one of the body's signs that it may be malnourished. Fatigue is also a sign of malnutrition, but in our society being tired is the norm. Individuals don't realize how tired they are until they are nourished and have more energy. The majority of signs of malnutrition don't occur until the body has been severely depleted.

Q: How can I follow my eating plan once I am discharged from the hospital (where I had support 24/7)?

A: Without constant support, it can be difficult to continue on your prescribed eating plan. Ideally, you will transition from inpatient treatment through the different levels of care (partial hospitalization and intensive outpatient) to outpatient. Ongoing support and working with a full treatment team is critical at this phase of treatment. You are trying to eat the prescribed amount of food, while your brain is telling you to restrict. Share with your treatment providers what your eating disorder voice is saying so they can help you begin to rewire your brain and the messages you are hearing.

CHAPTER 10

Treatment Protocols and
Higher Levels of Care

Five levels of care are available to individuals struggling with an eating disorder, depending on the intensity of their physiological, nutritional, and psychological needs: outpatient, intensive outpatient, partial hospitalization, residential, and inpatient care. The first level of care, outpatient, is the level of care that is the least restrictive and it is where most individuals who have eating disorders begin. The first part of this chapter will focus on the approach we take in providing outpatient care, as well as provide insight into the treatment team we put together and the treatment protocol we use. The rest of this chapter will discuss the remaining four levels of care and provide readers with what they should ask when seeking a Higher Level of Care (HLOC).

TREATMENT TEAM: TAKING A MULTIDISCIPLINARY APPROACH

One of the most important aspects of treating patients in an outpatient program is building a treatment team. Throughout this book, we have highlighted the complicated physiological, psychological, and nutritional issues that affect eating-disordered individuals. Since this is a multifaceted disease, we strongly advocate for a multidisciplinary treatment team to be put into place. Additionally, we highly recommend that each clinician on that team should have specialized experience and training in eating disorders. When patients are being treated at a level of care more intensive than outpatient, the clinicians typically have expertise in eating disorders. In our practices, our approach has been to take a multidisciplinary approach including professionals consisting of a medical doctor, a psychotherapist, a nutritionist/dietitian, and a psychiatrist when indicated. We think this is an ideal team and has led to our high success rate in treating patients.

RECOMMENDATIONS FOR THOSE SEEKING TREATMENT

There are many different treatment styles and matching the treatment to the patient is extremely important. For individuals who are seeking treatment for their eating disorder, we would recommend they identify a treatment team they feel comfortable with and can relate to. Another notable thing to look for when selecting a treatment team is identifying a clinician who is willing to collaborate in a team approach. Care will not be as comprehensive if there is only one clinician providing care. We do recognize that in the outpatient setting it is not always easy to find clinicians experienced in eating disorder treatment, especially in rural parts of the country and whose services are covered by the patient's insurance. However, for the best treatment outcome, there should be at least one clinician on the treatment team who has an expertise in eating disorder treatment.

Families will sometimes complain about the distance they have to travel for care. Would they be willing to travel if their child had cancer or would they prefer to have the treatment done by someone not as experienced in the care? The death rate for Anorexia Nervosa in the U.S. is 12 times higher than all other leading causes of death combined for the 15 - 24 age group.

OUTPATIENT TREATMENT PROTOCOL

The following chart depicts the treatment protocol we have in place at both of our practices.

Treatment Protocol

A multidisciplinary treatment team, including physician, psychotherapist dietitian/nutritionist, and psychiatrist (if indicated).

Initial evaluation including a medical exam, baseline blood work, nutrition assessment including MT and BCA, and psychological evaluation.

Devise an eating plan to initially stabilize the individual and then adjust intake to address nutritional status.

Weekly appointment with the psychotherapist and dietitian/nutritionist, monthly appointment with the physician.

Weekly Body Composition Analysis to assess the progress and guide treatment recommendations.

Initial Evaluation

The initial outpatient evaluation should include a medical, nutritional and psychological assessment. A comprehensive physical and medical exam includes blood work and an EKG; a psychological evaluation includes assessing the signs and symptoms of the eating disorder, as well as co-morbidities; the nutritional assessment includes baseline Metabolic Testing and Body Composition Analysis; and the psychiatric evaluation assesses for co-morbid conditions and medication management.

We would once again like to emphasize the importance of MT and BCA being part of our initial evaluation and strongly advocate for them to be normal protocol in any prescreening process. The data we obtain from these two tests are critical in helping us determine how severely the patient's body is malnourished. They minimize the chances of malnutrition being misdiagnosed, or worse, untreated.

Developing and Implementing an Outpatient Treatment Plan

Upon completion of the evaluation, the multidisciplinary team collaborates and develops an individualized treatment plan. At this time, the patient and family (if appropriate) are consulted and the treatment recommendations are discussed. If individuals are receiving services as an outpatient, they are typically seen one or more hours a week for an undetermined period of time to receive the support and treatment needed while continuing with "normal" life.

Initial treatment goals can include physical and psychological stabilization, nutritional rehabilitation, weight restoration (if needed), and normalization of blood work, as well as a significant decrease in symptoms including restricting, binging, and purging.

Throughout treatment, patients are typically seen weekly by the psychotherapist and nutritionist/dietitian, and monthly (or more frequently, if indicated) by the team's physician or their primary care physician. The frequency of psychiatry appointments depends on the clinician's practice. During this time, we also perform a weekly Body Composition Analysis on our patients and repeat the Metabolic Test if indicated. In addition, if outpatient groups are available, we encourage weekly attendance.

WHEN A HIGHER LEVEL OF CARE IS NECESSARY

If patients are unable to respond to the outpatient treatment, the treatment team then assesses them for a higher level of care. It is a difficult decision to seek a higher level of care; patients ask for **"one more chance"** to delay the inevitable. It is helpful to keep in mind that if individuals meet the criteria for a higher level of care, they will likely require that level of support until their symptoms stabilize and improve. While the decision to hospitalize is typically made by the treatment team, referrals can also be made by the individual or their family. Insurance companies have established criteria for each level of care, and an assessment or evaluation will be made by the treatment facility to determine appropriate care. Many factors are considered when determining level of care, including body weight, weight change, blood work abnormalities, self-harm risk, severity of symptoms, co-morbidities such as drugs and alcohol, support systems, home environment, previous treatment, and compliance with treatment.

Higher Level of Care Options

The following chart depicts the different options available when a higher level of care (HLOC) is necessary, their average length of stay, as well as their purpose.

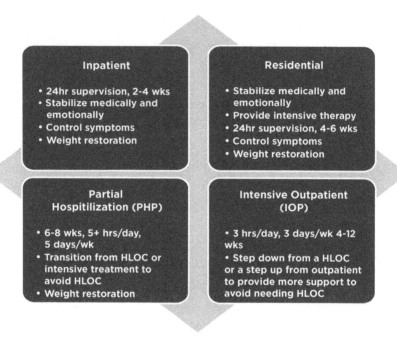

Figure 3. Higher Level of Care Options

Inpatient care is 24-hour supervision provided in a hospital setting. The majority of inpatient programs are in psychiatric hospitals. Inpatient care is used to stabilize the patient medically and emotionally, manage eating disorder behaviors and begin weight restoration. They are then transitioned to a lower level of care. An average length of stay is two to four weeks.

Residential treatment also provides 24-hour care, but is in a non-hospital setting. This level of care is designed for individuals who need more long-term structure and supervision to manage eating disorder symptoms and stabilize medically and emotionally, and begin weight restoration. An average length of stay is four to six weeks.

Partial hospitalization (PHP) is also referred to as day treatment. This level of care is a step down from more intensive treatment and also used when an individual needs more support than outpatient treatment. Treatment can be five to seven days a week and at least five hours a day. It is a group-based program, but patients have an individual therapist, nutritionist, and psychiatrist as part of the program. Weight restoration and management of eating disorder behaviors continue at this level of care. An average length of stay is six to eight weeks.

Intensive outpatient (IOP) is a step down from more intensive treatment and also used when more support in outpatient treatment is needed. This care is at least three days a week, three hours a day. It is group-based and requires the patient to have an outpatient team as well. An average length of stay is four to 12 weeks.

SELECTING A TREATMENT PROGRAM

We recommend patients who are considering a higher level of care ask the following questions:

- What types of medical monitoring and psychiatric care are provided?
- What is the patient-to-staff ratio?
- What is the average length of stay?
- What types of therapies are provided?
- How are patients transitioned from the program?
- Is there supervised overnight lodging for the partial hospitalization program?
- How many hours daily is the program and how many meals/snacks are included?

- What is my out-of-pocket cost?

- How are family and/or support individuals involved?

Insurance Coverage

Once a referral is made, the treatment facility will contact the insurance company to determine what benefits are available. It is very important when making arrangements for a higher level of care that you get confirmation of your out-of-pocket expense. Rates for residential or inpatient treatment can range from $1,000 to $2,000 a day. Rates for partial hospitalization range from $500 to $800 a day, and intensive outpatient programs are typically $300 to $500 a day. (Estimated amounts for 2015)

Questions and Answers for Higher Level of Care

Q: What happens when an individual needs treatment but does not have insurance?

A: Check to see if the patient meets the requirement for the state insurance plan. This can usually be done through their local Department of Social Services. For individuals who do not qualify for any type of coverage, some programs offer free treatment or scholarships.

Columbia Presbyterian in New York offers free 90-day programming as part of a research project. Mercy Ministries is a Christian treatment facility that provides free treatment. Manna Scholarship Fund, Moonshadows Spirit, Prazamana Foundation, Project Heal, Freed Foundation, and The Kirsten Haglund Foundation are some of the organizations that provide funding to families who are in need of help and can't afford treatment. These organizations all have websites and most of the application processes can be completed online.

Q: What if the individual does not feel sick enough for treatment?

A: An individual may not feel sick enough to go due to lack of insight, cognitive functioning and inherent ambivalence in eating disorders. They should have a thorough medical evaluation to determine if he or she needs higher level of care. In addition, the therapist, nutritionist, and psychiatrist should give their evaluations and recommendations. If higher level of care is recommended but delayed, the patient will likely deteriorate and there is a higher risk of the eating disorder becoming chronic. The longer a person is ill, the poorer the prognosis.

Q: When someone is discharged from the hospital, is it reasonable to expect him or her to be better?

A: Yes, but not fully recovered. The main purpose of hospitalization is to ensure that the individual is emotionally and physically safe and to stabilize symptoms. Some underlying emotional work has been done, but the majority of work occurs in the outpatient setting. Outpatient care is critical to successful recovery.

Q: What type of care can be provided at home?

A: The Maudsley Approach or Family Based Treatment (FBT) is a type of treatment that is done within the family. Below are websites with detailed explanations.

www.feast-ed.org
http://train2treat4ed.com/certifiedfbttherapists.html
http://maudsleyparents.org/providerlist.html
http://www.maudsleyparents.org/findtreatment.htm

"If you choose to take a homecare approach, you must recognize that you need daily vigilance and to stay committed for the duration—and not stop until it is done. The daily involvement, support, and perseverance are essential when caring for your loved one at home and it is very difficult since the situation is highly emotional with significant attention to detail and diligence being required."

– Allison's parents

CHAPTER 11

Recovery: Why It's Not a Linear Process

"I would encourage anyone who thinks they have a problem to get help. You don't know how much better your life can be until it's better. Even if you don't think you need it, give it a try and stick with it, because you don't know how poor your current quality of life is until you come out the other end and see how splendid it can be."

– Nicole

"I was so relieved when my daughter got out of the hospital. No more tears at mealtime, struggles with food, worrying if she was exercising or making herself throw up. We were finally past all of this. It was a real wake-up call when we realized she still worried if she was getting fat and had to still eat her safe foods. I didn't think we would have to keep going to treatment! I thought once she got out of the hospital she would be better."

– Patricia's father

RECOVERY IS A PROCESS

Recovery from an eating disorder is a process; it is very individualized and depends on many factors and dynamics. There are times when the patient is progressing and the eating disorder behaviors (e.g., purging, over-exercising, and restricting) and thoughts are minimal. There are also times when the behaviors are increased and patients seem vulnerable to a slip-up, but they still remain vigilant and are working hard in treatment. And then there are times when there is a relapse and a higher level of care is once again needed.

Recovery is not a linear process; there are many ups and downs. On good days the patient seems to take great strides in moving toward being symptom-free and emotionally stable; on not-so-good days slip-ups and relapses seem to be on the horizon.

Recovery involves many steps and there is no perfect recovery. Individuals with eating disorders have very high expectations for a perfect recovery but it is never a straightforward process; even the slightest relapse will make them feel like a failure. Families often think that after intensive treatment their sick family member should be completely better. While the individual may be better, it does not necessarily mean he or she is fully recovered. In fact, the real work may just be beginning. It is frustrating for families when the individual continues to show symptoms.

Outpatient treatment is a critical component of recovery where the majority of the treatment occurs. Clients who are transitioning from an inpatient setting may struggle with being thrown back into the "real world" where all the pressure and circumstances which initally led to the eating disorder are still present. Clients who are **"tired of treatment"** or think **"I can do this on my own"** are also at a higher risk of relapse. A comprehensive treatment team consist of (but not limited to) a physician, psychotherapist, dietitian/nutritionist, and psychiatrist (if indicated).

Although recovery is a complex and varied process, it does progress along three general stages: Early Recovery, Ongoing Recovery, and Fully Recovered. The ultimate goal is full recovery, in which a patient can live a life that is symptom free and emotionally harmonious.

EARLY RECOVERY STAGE

When individuals first enter treatment, the main focus is on emotional and physical stabilization. The initial focus is on controlling symptom use, weight restoration, and learning and using therapeutic skills to continue to control the behaviors. At this stage, patients will still struggle with a very strong eating disorder voice, typically telling them, *"You're fat, lazy, and weak," "If you eat what they tell you to, you will only get fat," "Don't trust them they only want you to get fat."* The use of therapeutic skills, such as those learned in cognitive behavioral therapy or dialectical behavioral therapy, helps them continue to move forward.

During this stage, patients will also struggle day-to-day with choices about food and exercise. They fear weight gain and have a strong desire to use unhealthy behaviors to compensate for eating foods they feel are unhealthy. This stage can last for several months or even years. Even when an individual has reached a recommended weight, he or she still struggles with a very strong eating disorder voice. The serotonin and dopamine pathways are still dysfunctional and may not ever completely normalize.

At-Risk for Relapse

Following intensive treatment (a higher level of care), it would be logical to assume patients would have an easier time doing what they need to do in order to take care of themselves. After all, they have had weeks or months to work on their treatment plan and they understand the consequences if they do not follow their treatment team's recommendations. However, individuals who were in a hospital or residential setting had support 24/7. Everyone there knew what they were thinking and feeling; they did not have to explain the eating disorder voice because it was understood.

Once discharged, patients are trying to cope with the eating disorder voice on their own 24/7. Ideally, an individual should transition from inpatient or residential to partial hospitalization and then outpatient. Stepping down from a higher level of care to a lesser one allows patients time to practice the skills they have acquired during treatment while still in a supportive setting.

Outpatient treatment, which is typically one to two hours a week, may be too little support initially for the individual who has been hospitalized. It is important to follow the treatment recommendations when being discharged to a lower level of care. Continued outpatient treatment is critical for successful long-term recovery. When the individual is trying to fight with the eating disorder voice, it is easy to become trapped into believing it again. The outpatient treatment team is there to help them understand what else is going on, as well as continuing to guide and reassure, helping them moving forward.

Emotional Stabilization

Co-morbidities, such as obsessive-compulsive disorder, anxiety disorder, or bipolar disorder to name a few, can make the recovery process more complicated. These need to be addressed at the same time as the eating disorder. Co-morbid psychiatric disorders strongly influence the dysfunctional brain mechanisms that regulate the serotonin and dopamine levels that may have initially predisposed them to eating disordered behavior.[1]

Therapeutically, the individual is beginning to understand the purpose of the eating disorder, the family dynamics that may have contributed to the development of the eating disorder, and their own personality traits that have predisposed them to eating problems, as well as the medical consequences. Many different types of therapeutic approaches can help them build skill sets, for example cognitive behavioral therapy, dialectical behavioral therapy, acceptance and commitment therapy, and mindfulness activities to cope with difficult situations. Emotion regulation is key to the recovery process.

Reassessing Level of Care

During early recovery, the individual continues to work with the outpatient treatment team, including a psychotherapist, nutritionist, physician, and at times, a psychiatrist. If eating disorder behaviors increase, the level of care the individual is receiving needs to be reassessed and this may lead to more intensive treatment. The level of care recommended is based on the physical condition and emotional state of the individual, as well as the symptom use. If individuals need more intensive care, it does not mean that they have "failed" treatment. It can be needed for many different reasons, including medical and/or emotional stabilization during the process, specialized treatment to address the co-morbid condition such as obsessive compulsive disorder (OCD), bipolar disorder, anxiety, or controlling symptom use, to name a few.

High-Risk Patients

For some, recovery can be the proverbial one step forward, two steps back. Deeply ingrained behaviors are hard to change. The process can take several years and many individuals do not get past the early recovery stage. These individuals are at very high risk of relapse and may need multiple hospitalizations to keep them safe. It is important to support them and try to help them see they are not failures. This is a patient population that feels whatever they do is not good enough and is very fearful of failure. The eating disorder voice is always reinforcing this. As much as it gets very tiresome and can be frustrating to continue to support loved ones through the process, it is critical to their recovery. When they hear, "I can't believe you aren't better yet," or "I can't believe you still do that [purge]," it just reinforces their belief that whatever they do is not good enough.

Multidisciplinary Team Approach

A multidisciplinary treatment team that specializes in eating disorder treatment is needed for recovery. If the individual is only working with a therapist, either food intake can be monitored or issues that need to be addressed in therapy can effectively be addressed, but not both. If patients are seeing only a nutritionist, they can work on the food, but accomplish very little therapeutically. If they are only seeing a physician, there may be focus on the food and symptoms, but very little or no focus on therapy. This is a very complex disease and needs a multidisciplinary treatment team approach.

ONGOING RECOVERY

Typically, recovery can take up to two to seven years. Some individuals may take much longer, depending on the co-morbidities present. The greater the co-morbidity, the more difficult it is to treat the eating disorder and the more chance that it can become chronic if not adequately managed. The cognitions and behaviors from the co-morbid disorder (e.g., OCD) make it more difficult to eat (increase in restrictive behavior), which causes the body to be malnourished, causing a decrease in the neurotransmitters including serotonin and dopamine that causes the comorbid disorder (the OCD) to worsen and makes the eating disorder more difficult to treat.[2]

There will be periods of time in the recovery process when the eating disorder voice is quieter and times when it is very loud. It is important to make sure patients realize that the eating disorder is always very quick to escalate.

Getting sick and not being able to eat for a few days will lead to a decrease in intake, which will decrease the neurotransmitter levels and lead to an increase in the obsessive thoughts. Individuals working on their recovery need to be hyper-vigilant about maintaining an adequate intake.

Intuitive Eating

Patients often want to begin to move toward more intuitive eating (eating when they are hungry and stopping when they are full). As much as this sounds like a normal progression, it is important to metabolically assess the patient first and make sure the body is at a normal metabolic rate. If an individual is still hypometabolic, the hunger cues will not trigger an adequate intake. The only way to determine if metabolism is normal is with Metabolic Testing.

Exercise

Exercise can be a healthy behavior for many in recovery. However, it is also very easy to trigger the exercise addiction. Each individual needs to be assessed. Going back to the gym can be very difficult for the compulsive exerciser. Working out on machines that display the amount of calories burned or other information should be avoided. Initially introducing activity that does not result in an endorphin high, such as walking, yoga, or participating in team sports, is a good way to start. The attitude toward exercise helps identify if it has potential to become problematic. We typically check in with patients, asking questions such as, "Do you feel you have to exercise to regulate your weight?" or "Do you enjoy the exercise you do?"

Body Image

Patients are always wondering when they will like their body. In our experience, body image is one of the last things to change. It seems to gradually shift, depending on how negative the body image initially was. Individuals who describe extreme body loathing will have difficultly ever embracing their body but may get to the point of acceptance or tolerance. Individuals who have felt "fat" and have struggled with body image may be able to embrace who they are as treatment progresses. It helps for patients to focus on how strong their bodies are or what their bodies are capable of doing to begin to appreciate them.

Trauma survivors often have more difficulty with body acceptance. The dopamine pathway also plays a part in how the body image changes. The dysregulation of the pathway leads to almost delusional thinking that the body is getting fatter with any food intake.

Overall, the treatment team focuses on the individual's behaviors and emotional and physical stability. At the same time, the individual is working on maintaining a healthy intake and balance in his or her life while continuing the therapeutic work that is needed.

FULLY RECOVERED

Individuals who struggle with eating disorders need to be hyper-vigilant about taking care of themselves in order to avoid relapse. We have seen individuals who are symptom-free and emotionally stable for more than ten years and then relapse. Many things that happen in life are unpredictable and can be difficult to handle emotionally. The eating disorder has been a coping mechanism that is protective when it comes to dealing with emotional pain. Individuals will describe initially losing their appetite and not eating at the same time they are dealing with depression. The decrease in intake causes a change in brain chemistry and the neurotransmitter levels which leads to an increase in obsessive thoughts. Patients describe hearing the eating disorder voice as if it never left. Patients often say it was not intentional, but just happened. Although not intentional, it is the same voice they heard when they were sick with the eating disorder.

As their bodies continue to heal from the eating disorder, individuals feel both emotionally and physically stronger. They are able to tolerate day-to-day events and not resort to eating disorder behaviors. Their response to a difficult situation is very different. Early in recovery, the desire to restrict or purge would be the automatic response. Fully recovered individuals have an ability to focus on the situation and determine how to best handle it.

Long-term recovery is also dependent upon periodic check-ups. When an individual has been weight restored and has been stable for at least six months, less frequent visits may be indicated. This needs to be mutually agreed upon by the treatment team and the patient. Since this is a patient population that struggles with abandonment issues, it is important for the treatment team to keep in mind that decreasing the frequency of their appointments may feel like rejection or abandonment. When this decision is a mutual one, they are less apt to feel abandoned. In our nutrition practices, patients eventually move to once every three to four months and may come in on an as-needed basis. An average length of treatment ranges from two to seven years.

From a physical perspective, recovery means the body has been weight restored; the metabolism is normal, and the body is no longer using its own protein stores to fuel itself. For females, there has been resumption of normal menses and the body is building and repairing tissue. Nutritionally, the individual is maintaining an adequate intake and not obsessing about food or weight. Exercise is something they enjoy doing, not what they feel they have to do.

Body Image

Body image is often the last thing to normalize. When patients are fully recovered, they are able to accept their body's natural body weight and are not focused on trying to lose weight. They are also able to accept that there are times in life (e.g., puberty, pregnancy, and menopause) when there will be shifts in body weight and embrace those times as part of what their body is naturally supposed to do. They are able to appreciate their body's abilities instead of focusing on what it cannot do or how it looks.

Exercise

In this stage, exercise is done for health and well-being. It may be that the individual who struggled with compulsive exercise might not be able to run competitively, but is able to hike and swim. Being aware that there are activities that can trigger a change in the serotonin and dopamine pathways is still very important. It is similar to the recovered alcoholic who has to avoid alcohol. Part of the self-care is being aware of how the body and brain responds to different activities.

The Importance of Daily Choices

In *Almost Anorexic,* author Jenni Schaefer writes about her recovery and how she views the eating disorder as the cliff.[2] She describes choices she makes every day as moving her closer to the cliff or further away. If she picks a diet soda or a salad for a meal because it has fewer calories, she is taking a step to move closer to the cliff. If she chooses to chew sugar-free gum to postpone hunger, she is moving closer to the cliff's edge. If she decides to take a casual walk instead of a run, knowing that she would spend more calories running, she is moving further from the edge. She describes the daily choices that face those struggling with an eating disorder as choices that are critical to their recovery.

Kate's Story

Kate, a former patient who had been in recovery for five years, started training for a marathon. She had always been an athlete and loved to run. She knew the training might trigger eating disorder thoughts but still wanted to try. Kate was able to train and run the marathon while still taking care of herself. The more she explored what was helpful and what wasn't, Kate was able to realize going to a gym was very high risk for her. Working out on machines that displayed the number of calories burned triggered her eating disorder voice. She enrolled in a CrossFit gym and found it to be the perfect fit. She was exercising with a group of people and the type of exercise was focused on strength. She didn't have to think about what the next activity would be because it was all preplanned, and the workout was finished in an hour.

Acceptance of Self

Individuals who struggle with an eating disorder typically are perfectionistic. As they progress in the recovery process, they move toward more acceptance of their imperfections, embracing who they are as an individual.

Belief that they are "good enough" just the way they are is part of being fully recovered.

> *"I have days where I compare my intake to those around me (I have to eat a lot!), and get down that my body sometimes gets tired and I know that I have to take a step back and get some rest. When I encounter days like the aforementioned, I know I have two choices: I can 1) chose to be overcome by comparison and negativity, or 2) chose to give my body what it needs and remember that my identity is not determined by those around me."*
>
> *– Colleen*

RESILIENCY

Resiliency is a key to a successful recovery. There will be many times when slip-ups or relapses happen, but the more resilient individuals are, the more determined they are to keep moving forward. It has been our experience that the more ego-strength or sense-of-self individuals have, the further they are able to go in the recovery process. Unconditional and ongoing support is critical for patients working on their recovery. They know if they relapse they are able to reach out for help much sooner because they know they will be supported. They do not fear that someone will think they are a failure.

The sooner patients are able to get the support they need to get back on track, the less influence the eating disorder voice will have on them. Individuals who have co-morbidities may be less resilient, not because they are not trying but because when the individual relapses, the co-morbidity (e.g., OCD, bipolar, depression) will also be affected. Both are affected by the dysregulation of the serotonin and dopamine pathways, which is exacerbated by eating disorder behaviors and malnutrition. However, becoming more resilient is a tangible, significant goal for our patients, especially since it can lead to a sustained recovery.

Questions and Answers for Relapse and Recovery

Q: What if my adolescent child says she isn't getting anything out of treatment?

A: It is not unusual for adolescents to be in treatment because their parents insist they get help. If this is the case, the child will often make treatment difficult and unbearable, hoping the parents will give in and allow them to discontinue. Although the expectation is that once your child starts treatment, things will improve, unfortunately things often appear worse before they get better. The decision to discontinue treatment should be a mutual decision between the treatment team, patient, and family if appropriate. Individuals ambivalent about their recovery often want to discontinue treatment when feeling uncomfortable.

Q: Are there alternative therapies that can be helpful in recovery?

A: In addition to cognitive behavioral therapy and relational therapy, some other types of treatment include, but are not limited to: dialectical behavioral therapy, internal family systems (IFS), eye movement desensitization reprocessing (EMDR), emotion freedom technique, art therapy, movement therapy, yoga, journaling, psychodrama, and neuro-feedback. A combination of many different therapies helps patients progress in their recovery.

Q: What are some things I can do to enhance my recovery?

A: Daily, you make choices to enhance your recovery. Doing what you want to do because you enjoy it, not because you can burn more calories, and selecting something you want to eat because you like it instead of choosing something else because it is lower in calories are examples of ways to strengthen your recovery. Self-care, including yoga and/or meditation, helps keep you present, which is also critical to your recovery. Taking time for yourself and keeping balance in your life will help strengthen your recovery.

Q: Will I ever be able to run like I used to?

A: The answer to this is that it is individualized. Some people are able to introduce running back into their life and enjoy it, while others are not able to because it triggers the exercise addiction. Work with your treatment team and re-introduce activity gradually. You will recognize if the activity is triggering the addiction. It is critical that you let your team know right away so they can help you avoid relapse. It is key to properly fuel your body for the activity to maintain nutritional balance.

Q: How do I convince someone I care about to get treatment when she is in denial?

A: It is very difficult for you to watch someone struggle and not be able to help them. As clinicians, we often keep each other in check by reminding ourselves that we cannot work any harder than the patient is working. When an individual is in denial or refusing to get help, it is important for you to take care of yourself. Working with a therapist will help you identify ways to be supportive of the individual, but not enable them.

CHAPTER 12

Final Thoughts: From Small Steps to Milestones

"I have truly gained freedom. I learned that my identity was not in my eating disorder and that I couldn't allow this disorder to control my life. Although my body had been healing a little over a year, my mind was leaning toward eating disorder thoughts. I've realized that I can choose freedom from these thoughts, when I just surrender them and remember that I wasn't created to feel this way, to live in darkness. It's an everyday choice to recover—it goes far beyond the physical recovery."

- Colleen

Eating disorders do not have to be a lifelong struggle. With adequate support and treatment, recovery is possible. As discussed in the previous chapter, recovery is a very complicated process, but when finally achieved and sustained, it will have a profound effect on the life of someone who has struggled with an eating disorder. This last chapter will include our final thoughts regarding recovery and how taking small steps can lead to sustained recovery resulting in lifelong milestones.

SUSTAINED RECOVERY: FROM OUR PERSPECTIVE

There are many components to recovery: normal metabolic rate, body composition showing muscle, fat, fat-free mass and phase angle all within normal ranges, normal menstruation, healthy energy, and absence of the eating disorder voice. Individuals are no longer obsessing about what to eat and when to exercise; they are able to develop a normal relationship with food and eat intuitively to meet their physical needs. Exercise becomes an activity they enjoy doing and choose to do when they want to, not when they feel they have to.

Accepting their body and embracing who they are is also a critical component to long-term recovery. They are finally able to set limits and boundaries with individuals and not apologize for it. As clinicians, we look for quantifiable data— often obtained through Metabolic Testing and Body Composition Analysis—as well as assessing information gathered from other members of the patient's treatment team when determining whether or not a patient can be deemed "fully recovered."

While we analyze quantitative data, we also seek qualitative data. For example, when a 50-year-old patient brings in a photo of herself in a bathing suit while on vacation and is excited because it is the first time she has ever worn a bathing suit, we pay close attention. The data we had already obtained on this patient— whether it was a normal metabolic rate, or one of the other measurable data outlined above—is significant in determining whether or not she is sustaining her recovery. But the qualitative data we see, when she disclosed how high her comfort level was in wearing a bathing suit for the first time, is equally valuable. It allows us to examine the effect sustaining recovery is having on her life.

This type of feedback, which is often very intimate and personal, signifies that a foundation has been put in place, allowing a patient to put an eating disorder permanently into the past. The following illustrates a small example of the milestones we have collected over the years from the work we do.

YOU CAN'T DO ANYTHING DIFFERENT, UNTIL YOU SEE IT DIFFERENTLY

Our overall philosophy in working with eating disorders is: *"You can't do anything different until you see it differently."* As clinicians, this philosophy is infused into our practices and influences us to incorporate Metabolic Testing and Body Composition Analysis into our treatment protocol. It drives us to break away from numbers on a scale and instead to measure health from the inside. We also try to impart this way of thinking to our patients so they're not relying on numbers on a scale when gauging their recovery. Instead, they're tuned in to changes in their bodies, as well as the way they think about themselves.

A grandmother looking at her first grandchild. Thankful her now recovered daughter was able to have a healthy pregnancy and can experience the joys of motherhood.

A patient who has not had her menstrual cycle in over ten years reports she is finally eating enough to have her menses start.

A patient who had a cardiac arrest while at an impatient unit. She took ten medical leave of absences before she was able to complete college, is now a happy mother of three healthy children.

A 23-year-old male who struggled with Anorexia since age 14 is now healthy and a professional entertainer.

A patient reports she is thrilled because she just beat her own personal record in a college cross country race, and was able to do it with her new and "bigger" body.

A 28-year-old who has been hospitalized with Anorexia, more than half her life, recently graduated from college, is living independently, and has job in the human service field.

A 35-year-old whose initial goal when first seeking treatment was "I just want to live to graduate from college." She is now working for NIH in cancer research and a mother of two beautiful children.

The following testimonials, collected over the years, provide examples illustrating how our patients have benefited from this philosophy. We want to end this book with their words—words that describe recovery in reflective and profound ways.

"My journey hasn't been straightforward, but it has resulted in lasting changes: my bones are no longer brittle, I am closer to my family, I have developed a loving

and healthy relationship with my husband, and I main-
tained a healthy pregnancy that led to the birth of my
beautiful son. While I am still stubborn and at times my
stubbornness hinders my recovery, I now try to invest my
energy towards my life, not against it."

– Julie

"Recovery is... feeling my life! Breathing and taking it all in.
Facing my fears. Being brave. Allowing myself to accept
the blessings that are all around me. Owning my story
and taking pride in who I am."

– Jen

"The only person who could ever truly understand me
was myself, so I thought. Now, I consider myself more of
a realist. I still exercise daily and still hope to become a
journalist of some description, but I hold those aspects
of my life to a realistic standard. In essence, I just don't
bite off more than I can chew. My social life, too, has benefited from this mindset. I no longer have these unrealistic expectations of how my friends should be and rather
accept them for who they are. They are my friends, after
all, and they know more about me than I think I know
about myself."

– Soren

"Today when I look at how far I have come, I often cry. I
feel so much sorrow and empathy for the person I was.
She is still part of me, but not as someone I identify myself
as. She walks with me as a reminder of how far I have
come. Today I am doing things I never thought possible.
I own my business. My marriage has been saved, and
my relationship with my children is strong. It has been a

very emotionally challenging journey. It's a journey that is ongoing. It's so important to open yourself up and get the assistance and guidance you need. I could not have made the changes I've made without the help of others."

– Jeanette

"When I had an eating disorder, I lived in a box where everything was controlled and disciplined. I didn't look far into the future and I didn't have to deal with my emotions too much—I numbed them by not eating. Life was simpler in a lot of ways, but it was two-dimensional. Today, two-and-a-half years later, life is much richer and more complex. I had to relearn boundaries and how to express myself appropriately, now that I don't use my disorder to numb myself. I am now starting to expand my social activities; I am getting married and am excited about the future. Some days it's still a challenge, but the rewards are great!"

– Louise

"My thoughts about myself are much more kind, I can acknowledge my flaws and mistakes without overwhelming shame, and I can embrace my strengths and successes. One of my fears was that everyone else would be happy with my recovery and I would be miserable. I learned it's a common fear. When I had my eating disorder, my life was very small but very chaotic. Now I have so much more going on in my life and I'm much happier with my bigger life."

– Kadee

"Today, my friends make up a huge portion of my life, whereas before, they remained out of convenience (the

deepest level of connection I could maintain given my intense devotion the omnipotent Food). I would love to say I know what I want to do with my life next year, after graduation, or once I reach the dreaded adulthood, but I am confident in my abilities, including being able to see past the details, if only a little. I am unafraid of the future, be it planning my future or following the path of self-discovery a little further. I can look at my plans for today, for tomorrow, for forever, and be satisfied with that which I know and even more contented with the great anticipation of that which I don't. But of all the things I've gained in recovery, more things than I could ever have hoped or dreamed to have attained, relearning who I am has been the most rewarding. I feel blessed to be able to look at life with such positivity and with such possibility, after having come so close to losing my life, and myself, entirely."

- Nicole

NOTES

Introduction

1. P. F. Sullivan. "Mortality in Anorexia Nervosa," *American Journal of Psychiatry* 152, no. 7 (1995): 1073-74.

2. S. Crow, C. Peterson, S. Swanson, N. Raymond, S. Specker, E. D. Eckert, & J. E. Mitchell. "Increased mortality in bulimia nervosa and other eating disorders," *American Journal of Psychiatry* 166 (2009: 1342-46.

Chapter 1

1. "Minnesota Starvation Experiment," *Wikipedia*, last modified October 10, 2014, http://en.wikipedia.org/wiki/Minnesota_Starvation_Experiment.

2. Kathleen Mahan L. and Sylvia Escott-Stump. *Krause's Food & Nutrition Therapy* (St. Louis: Saunders Elsevier, 2007) 67.

3. "Consequences of Eating Disorders," Eating Problems Service, retrieved from http://www.eatingproblems.org/epseffect.html. L.J.Hoffer and P.J. Jones, "Clinical Nutrition: 1. Protein-energy malnutrition in the inpatient. CMAJ Nov 13 2001;165 (10): 1345 - 1349

4. "Starvation Response," *Wikipedia*, last modified October 7, 2014, http://enwikipedia.org/wiki/starvation_mode.

5. Carlos M. Grillo and James Mitchell. *Treatment of Eating Disorders,* (New York: NY Guilford Press, 2010) 68.

6. James E. Mitchell and Scott Crow. "Medical Complications of Anorexia Nervosa and Bulimia Nervosa," *Current Opinion Psychiatry* 19 (2006): 438-443.

7. S. Grinspoon, E. Thomas, S. Pitts, E. Gross, D. Mickley, K. Miller, D. Herzog, and A. Klibanski. "Prevalence and Predictive Factors for Regional Osteopenia in Women with Anorexia Nervosa," *Annals of Internal Medicine* 133, no. 10 (2000): 790-794.

8. James M. Greenblatt. *Answers to Anorexia: A Breakthrough Nutritional Treatment That Is Saving Lives,* (North Branch: MN Sunrise River Press, 2010) 14, 21, 29 & 156.

9. M. Maine, B. Hartman McGilley, and D. W. Bunnell. *Treatment of Eating Disorders: Bridging the Research-Practice Gap* (London, Burlington, San Diego: Elsevier, 2010) 96, 102.

10. Ibid.

11. Ralph E. Carson. *The Brain Fix,* (Deerfield Beach: Health Communications, 2010) 37-37.

12. W.H. Kaye, G. K. Frank, U. F. Bailer, and S. E. Henry. "Neurobiology of anorexia nervosa: Clinical implications of alterations of the function of serotonin and other neuronal systems," *International Journal of Eating Disorder* 37 (2005): S15-S19.

13. Maine M., B. Hartman McGilley, and D. W. Bunnell, *Treatment of Eating Disorders,* 96 & 102.

14. Greenblatt, James M., *Answers to Anorexia,* 14, 21, 29 & 156.

15. Charles F. Saladino. "The Efficacy of Bioelectrical Impedance Analysis (BIA) in Monitoring Body Composition Changes During Treatment of Restrictive Eating Disorder Patients" *Journal of Eating Disorders 2014, 2:34.*

Chapter 2

1. W. H. Kaye, J. Fudge, and M. Paulus. "New Insights into Symptoms and Neurocircuit Function of AN," *Nature Reviews Neuroscience* 10 (2009): 573-84.

2. Martha M. Levine, Peaslee and Richard L. Levine. "Psychiatric Medication: Management, Myths, and Mistakes," (2010) in Maine, M., Hartman McGilley, B., and Bunnell, D.W., *Treatment of Eating Disorders, Bridging the Research-Practice Gap* (London, Burlington, San Diego: Elsevier, 2010) 111-126.

3. L. Hill, D. Dagg, M. Levine, L. Smolak, S. Johnson, S. Stotz, and N. Little. *Family Eating Disorders Manual: Guiding Families Through the Maze of Eating Disorders* (The Center for Balanced Living, Worthington: Ohio, 2012): 83-4.

Chapter 3:

1. Y. Schultz. "The Basis of Direct and Indirect Calorimetry and their Potentials," *Diabetes/Metabolism Reviews* 11, no. 4, (1995): 383-408. Retrieved from http://www.ncbi.nlm.nih.gov/myncbi/collections

2. Monitoring Metabolic Status:Predicting Decrements in Physiological and Cognitive performance, 2004 by Committee on Metabolic Monitoring for military Field Applications, Standing Committee on Military Nutrition Research, Chapter 3, Monitoring Overall Physical Status to Predict Performance; Laboratory Methods, p. 8, National Academic Press US

3. Rifat Latifi and Stanley J. Dudrick. *The Biology and Practice of Current Nutritional Support*, (Georgetown: MD Landes Bioscience, 2003) 5.

4. E.F. Coyle. "Substrate Utilization During Exercise in Active People," *American Journal of Clinical Nutrition* 61 (1995): 968S-79S.

5. L. Scalfi, M Marra, A. Caldara, E. Silvestri, and F. Contaldo. "Changes in Bioimpedance Analysis after Stable Refeeding of Undernourished Anorexic Patients," *International Journal of Obesity & Related Metabolic Disorders: Journal of the International Association for the Study of Obesity* 23, no. 2 (1999): 133-137.

Chapter 4

1. P. F. Sullivan. "Mortality in Anorexia Nervosa," *American Journal of Psychiatry* 152 (1995): 1073-1074.

2. "Eating Disorders 101 Guide: A Summary of Issues, Statistics, and Resources," *The Renfrew Center Foundation for Eating Disorders,* 2003, http://www.renfrew.org.

3. James M. Greenblatt. *Answers to Anorexia A Breakthrough Nutritional Treatment That Is Saving Lives,* (North Branch: MN Sunrise River Press, 2010) 19.

4. "Eating Disorders 101 Guide," *The Renfrew Center Foundation for Eating Disorders.*

5. National Eating Disorder Association, 2005, http://www. NationalEatingDisorders.org

6. A. T. Faje, P. K. Fazeli, K. K. Miller, D. K. Katzman, S. Ebrahimi, H. Lee, N. Mendes, D. Snelgrove, E. Meenaghan, M. Misra, and A. Klibanski. "Fracture Risk and Areal Bone Mineral Density in Adolescent Females with Anorexia Nervosa," *Internal Journal of Eating Disorders* 47 (2014): 458-466.

7. Minuchin, S., Rosman, S., and Baker, B. L. *Psychosomatic Families: Anorexia Nervosa in Context,* (Cambridge: MA Harvard University Press, 1978).

8. C. Fairburn, Z. Cooper, H. A. Doll. "Risk Factors for Anorexia Nervosa," *Archives of General Psychiatry* 56, no. 5 (1999): 468-476.

9. M. A. Kalarchian, M. Marcus, and A. Courcoulas. "Eating Problems after Bariatric Surgery," *Eating Disorder Review* 19, no. 4 (2008).

Chapter 5

1. American Psychiatric Association. *Disorders,* 5th ed. (text rev., Washington, DC: American Psychological Association, 2014).

2. Philip S. Mehler and Arnold E. Andersen. *Eating Disorders: A Guide to Medical Care and Complications,* (Baltimore, MD: John Hopkins University Press, 2010) 111-123, 135, 173-177.

3. Ibid.

4. Ibid.

5. National Eating Disorders Association, 2005, http://www. NationalEatingDisorders.org.

6. Mehler, Phillip S., *Eating Disorders,* 111-123, 135, 173-177.

7. Ibid.

8. Ibid.

9. W. H. Kaye, G. K. Frank, U. F. Bailer, and S. E. Henry. "Neurobiology of Anorexia Nervosa: Clinical Implications of Alterations of the Function of Serotonin and other Neuronal Systems," *International Journal of Eating Disorders* 37, no. 10 (2005): S15-S19.

10. S. A. Swanson, S. J. Crow, D. LeGrange, J. Swendsen, K. R. Merikangas. "Prevalence and Correlates of Eating Disorders in Adolescents: Results from the National Comorbidity Survey Replication-Adolescent Supplement," *Archives of General Psychiatry* 24, no. 2 (2001): 714-723.

11. Charles F. Saladino. "Is Bioelectrical Impedance Analysis (BIA) Efficacious in Monitoring Body Composition Changes During Treatment of Restrictive Eating Disorder Patients?" *Renfrew Perspectives*, (2012): 15-17.

Chapter 6

1. National Eating Disorders Association, 2005, http://www.NationalEatingDisorders.org.

2. "Binge-Eating Disorder," Mayo Clinic, April 3, 2012, http://www.mayoclinic.org/diseases-conditions/binge-eating-disorder/basics.

Chapter 7

1. Susan Solenberger. "Exercise and Eating Disorders: A 3-year Inpatient Hospital Record Analysis," *Eating Behaviors* 2, no. 2 (2001): 151-168.

2. J. C. Carter, E. Blackmore, K. Sutandar-Pinnock, and D. B. Woodside. "Relapse in Anorexia Nervosa: A Survival Analysis," *Psychology Medicine* 34, no. 4 (2004): 71-679.

3. "Compulsive Exercise: Are You Overdoing It? Frisch,R. New England Journal of Medicine, 1980. accessed from http://teens.webmd.com/compulsive-exercise, February 2014.

4. R. M. Calogero and K. N. Pedrotty-Stump. "Incorporating Exercise into Eating Disorder Treatment and Recovery," In Margo Maine, et al., *Treatment of Eating Disorders: Bridging the Research-Practice Gap*, (London, Burlington, San Diego: Elsevier, 2010) 435.

5. Carolyn Costin. *The Eating Disorder Sourcebook* (Los Angeles: Lowell House, 1999).

6. O. L. Miller and J. Spies-Gans. "Disorderly Conduct," *The Harvard Crimson*, 2014, http://www.thesportinmind.com/articles/addicted-to-exercise-when-too-much-exercise-might-be-harmful/.

7. W. H. Kaye, J. Fudge, and M. Paulus. "New Insights into Symptoms and Neurocircuit Function of Anorexia Nervosa," *Nature Reviews Neuroscience* 10 (2009): 573-584. doi: 10.1038/nrn2682.

8. "Addiction," *Integrative Psychiatry*, 2014, http://www.integrativepsychiatry.net/addiction_recovery.html.

9. Ralph E. Carson. *The Brain Fix,* (Deerfield Beach: Health Communications, 2012) 26.

10. Ibid.

11. Margo Mountjoy et al, "The IOC consensus statement: beyond the Female Athlete Triad - Relative Energy Deficiency in Sports (RED-S)," British Journal of Sports Medicine 2014; 48:491-497.

12. "Female Athlete Triad," Kids Health, http://kidshealth.org/teen/food_fitness/sports/triad.html.

13. "Menstruation and the Menstrual Cycle," The National Women's Health Information Center, 2012, http://womenshealth.gov/publications/our-publications/fact-sheet/menstruation.html.

14. "Osteoporosis," National Institutes of Health, 2006, http://www.niams.nih.gov/Health_Info/Osteoporosis/default.asp.

Chapter 8

1. S. Crow, C. Peterson, S. Swanson, N. Raymond, S. Specker, E. D. Eckert, and J. E. Mitchell. "Increased Mortality in Bulimia Nervosa and other Eating Disorders," *American Journal of Psychiatry* 166 (2009): 1342-1346.

2. American Psychiatric Association. *Disorders,* 5th ed. (text rev., Washington, DC: American Psychological Association, 2014).

Chapter 9

1. USDA, Center for Nutrition Policy and Promotion. *Dietary Guidelines for Americans* (Washington, DC: National Academy Press, 2010).

2. Helen A. Picciano and Mary Francis Guthrie. *Human Nutrition* (St. Louis, MO: Mosby, 1995).

3. "Leading Sources of Protein, Fats, Carbohydrates and Fiber," USDA National Nutrient Database for Standard Reference, 2014, http://ndb.nal.usda.gov/.

4. R. Estruch, E. Ros, J. Salas-Salvado et al. "Primary Prevention of Cardiovascular Disease with a Mediterranean Diet," *New England Journal of Medicine* 368 (2013): 1279-90.

5. Aseem Malhotra. "Saturated Fats is not the Major Issue," *British Medical Journal* 347 (2013): f6340.

6. Jennifer Andrews. "Sickness Caused by Lack of Fats and Oils in the Diet," Diet and Nutrition, Livestrong, 2013, http://www.lifestrong.com/fats.

7. Blake Graham. "Essential Fatty Acid Deficiency-Signs & Symptoms, Treating Vs. Testing," ProHealth, 2009, http://www.prohealth.com/library/showarticle.cfm?libid=7564.

8. "Dietary Guidelines for Americans," USDA and USHHS, 2010, http://www.hhs.gov.

9. J. L. Slavin. "Position of the American Dietetic Association: Health Implications of Dietary Fiber," *Journal of the American Dietetic Association* 108 (2008): 1716-1731.

10. FAO/WHO/UNU Joint Report. *Energy and Protein Requirements*, Technical Rep Series 724 (Geneva, Switzerland: World Health Organization, 1985).

11. Philip S. Mehler and Arnold E. Andersen. *Eating Disorders: A Guide to Medical Care and Complications*, (Baltimore, MD: The John Hopkins University Press, 2010) 111.

12. James M., Greenblatt. *Answers to Anorexia: A Breakthrough Nutritional Treatment That Is Saving Lives*, (North Branch: MN Sunrise River Press, 2010) 156.

13. M. Garaulet, P. Gomez-Abellan, J. J. Alburquerque-Bejar, Y. C. Lee, J. M. Ordovas, and F. A. J. L. Scheer. "Timing of Food Intake Predicts Weight Loss Effectiveness," *International Journal of Obesity* 37 (2013): 604-611.

Chapter 11

1. K. Willis. " DSM-5 and Eating Disorders," *Gurze Eating Disorders Resource Catalogue*, 2014, http://www.edcatalogue.com/dsm-5-eating-disorders/.

2. Jennifer J. Thomas and Jenni Schaefer. *Almost Anorexic* (Center City, Minnesota: Hazelden, 2013).

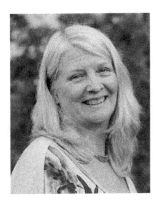

CAROLYN HODGES CHAFFEE, MS, RDN, CEDRD is the founder and director of the Upstate New York Eating Disorder Service, Nutrition Clinic and Sol Stone Center; serving over 8000 patients since 1990. She helped design and implement the eating disorder program at Cornell University, serving over 400 patients annually. She was the Nutrition Consultant to the 2004 women's Olympic crew team. Learn more about her work at www.unyed.com.

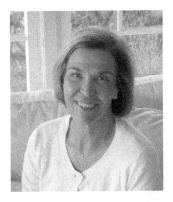

ANNIKA KAHM, MS, has been treating eating disorders for over thirty years. She is the founder and director of Medical Nutrition Therapy in Stamford, Connecticut. Annika is the co-author of three books and numerous papers. Learn more about her work at www.annikakahm.com.

INDEX

Activity Disorder. *See* compulsive exercise.

Actual Resting Energy Expenditure (AREE), 22, 24, 25

Amenorrhea, 7, 24, 4q4
    and compulsive exercise, 68, 69, 70, 73

Amino acids, 13, 88

Anabolism, 21

Anemia, 5, 71

Anorexia Athletica, 64

Anorexia Nervosa, 3, 7, 8, 9, 21, 31–32, 44, 55, 63, 66, 67, 76, 77, 81
    and denial, 36
    at a younger age, 38–39
    characteristics of, 32
    contribution of serotonin to traits of, 9, 35, 42
    current trends in, 36–39
    identification of, 33–34
    in bariatric patients, 37–38
    incidence rate of, 33
    malnutrition in, 32, 33, 38, 39, 40, 42
    mortality rate for, 33, 99
    neurological and psychological changes and complications of, 35–36
    other complaints in, 34–35
    physiological changes and complications of, 34
    questions and answers for, 41–42
    self-induced vomiting in, 38
    stomach complaints in, 34
    usefulness of MT and BCA in, 36, 39–40
    warning signs of, 33–34

Anxiety, 11, 12, 13, 14f, 16, 17, 35, 39, 44, 48, 49, 51, 55, 56, 57, 60, 63, 68, 69, 76, 81, 94, 110
    reduction of, 12, 16, 17, 27, 44, 51, 63
    when normal eating resumes, 17
    Atypical Anorexia Nervosa, 75, 76, 77, 78–79

Binge Eating Disorder (BED), 3, 22, 53–54, 77–78, 81
    as physiological response from Anorexia Nervosa, 55
    and dieting, 54–55, 56, 59, 60
    and eating disorder voice, 54
    at a younger age, 54
    causes of, 54–55, 60
    differences from compulsive overeating, 60
    identification of, 55–56
    neurological and psychological changes and complications of, 56 – 57
    physiological changes and complications of, 56
    prevalence of, 55
    questions and answers for, 60–61
    treatment protocols for, 59
    usefulness of MT and BCA in, 57–59
    warning signs of, 56

Body checks, 32

Body Composition Analysis (BCA), 9, 10, 19–20, 22, 23, 26–27, 27f, 29, 30, 34, 36, 39, 40, 41, 42, 49, 50, 57, 58, 59, 71, 72, 79, 81, 82, 83, 87, 90, 91, 92, 94, 95, 97, 100, 120
    questions and answers for, 29–30

Body fat, 6, 26, 30, 69, 72, 79, 85, 89, 91
    loss of, 6
    use during starvation, 6
Body mass index (BMI), 30, 38, 79
Bone loss, 6-7, 35, 69, 70, 71, 73, 74
Brain chemistry, change in, 11, 17, 33, 35, 54, 65–67, 113
    when body is underfed, 13–14

Breakfast, importance of, 51, 58, 60–61, 83, 92-93

Bulimia Nervosa, 3, 8, 21, 37, 43–44, 63, 66, 76, 77, 81

    binge eating in, 44, 46, 51

    cardiac complications in, 47

    case study, 48–49

    common complaints, 47

    compensatory behaviors in. *See* Bulimia Nervosa, purging.

    dehydration in, 50, 52

    dental problems in, 47

    diuretic use, complications from, 47

    diuretic use in, 44, 46, 50

    excessive exercise in, 44, 45, 46, 50

    gastrointestinal reflux symptoms in, 45

    laxative use, complications from, 45, 47

    laxative use in, 44, 47, 50

    mood instability and anxiety, 48

    neurological and psychological changes and complications of, 47–48

    perceived loss of control in, 44

    physiological changes and complications of, 47–48

    purging, 21, 22, 43, 44—46, 47, 48—49, 50, 51, 52, 78, 82, 86, 101, 107, 113

    purging, fallout from, 44–45, 47

    questions and answers for, 51–52

    self-induced vomiting in, 44, 45, 46, 47, 50

    serotonin and dopamine levels, 47–48

    shame, 43, 45, 51

    suicide risk, 48

    throat complications from, 45

    usefulness of MT and BCA in, 50

    warning signs of, 46

Carbohydrates, 13, 14f, 15, 36, 41, 87, 88, 89, 90, 95

    as source of blood glucose, 89, 90

    complex, 15, 90

    simple, 90

Carbohydrate restriction, 13, 14f, 14–15, 36
Catabolic state, 1, 2, 4, 5, 21, 25, 26, 33, 40, 48, 49, 50, 57, 68, 72, 78, 82, 87, 92
    diagnosis of, 24–25
Catabolism, 21, 25
Celiac disease, 7, 95–96
Compulsive exercise, 9, 22, 45, 50, 62–63, 64, 113, 115
    and amenorrhea, 69
    and anxiety, 63, 69
    and control, 63
    and depression, 69
    and eating disorder voice, 62–63, 67–68
    brain changes due to, 65–66
    cardiac complications in, 69
    definition of *too much* exercise, 73
    fatigue, 68, 70
    guilt in, 63
    identification of, 64
    in Anorexia Nervosa, 33
    in Bulimia Nervosa, 50
    insomnia, 69
    neurological and psychological changes and complications of, 69–70
    physiological changes and complications of, 68–69
    questions and answers for, 73–74
    social isolation, 69
    usefulness of MT and BCA for, 71–72
    warning signs of, 68
Control, 11–12, 16
    loss of, 11, 12, 17, 35, 44, 53, 54
    of anxiety, 76
    of food, 12, 46
    of life by eating disorder, 15, 119, 123
    sense of, 12, 59
    weight control, 54, 63, 64

Cortisol, 67, 68
Denial, 10, 25, 35, 36, 90, 119–120
    in Anorexia Nervosa, 36
    in compulsive exercising, 72
Depression, 2, 11, 13, 14f, 16, 114, 116
exercise as treatment for, 62
    in Anorexia Nervosa, 35
    in Binge Eating Disorder, 56
    in Bulimia Nervosa, 49
    in Compulsive Exercise, 69
    in OSFED, 81
Diabetes mellitus. *See* Diabetes, Type 2.
Diabetes, Type 1, 48, 49
Diabetes, Type 2, 7, 37, 56, 81, 85
Disordered eating, 3
Distorted body image, 8, 32–33, 35, 48, 66, 112–113, 114
Dopamine, 9, 13, 47, 65, 66, 110, 111, 113, 114, 115, 117
Dysfunctional exercise. *See* compulsive exercise.
Early recovery stage, 108 –111
Eating disorders, 1, 2
    and malnutrition, 1, 3, 8
    at-risk for relapse, 109–110
    development of, 3
    emotional stabilization, 110
    environment, 9
    evolution of, 9
    genetics, 9
    guilt, 9, 14
    hiding of, 20
    high-risk patients, 110
    impact on metabolism, 21
    importance of daily choices, 115
    multidisciplinary team approach, 110
    prevalent complications of, 6–8
    reassessing level of care, 110

relation to obsessive-compulsive thoughts, 12–13

stabilization focus, 108

Eating Disorders, Not Otherwise Specified (EDNOS), 76, 77

Eating disorder voice, 11–12, 15, 17, 18

after fully recovered, 113, 115

and resiliency, 116

evolution from obsessive-compulsive thinking, 12–13

in Anorexia Nervosa, 32, 39

in Binge Eating Disorder, 54, 55

in Compulsive Exercise, 62–63, 67–68

in early recovery, 108–109, 111

in ongoing recovery, 112

in OSFED, 80

in sustained recovery, 120

Endorphins, 62–63, 65–66, 74, 112

Exercise addiction. *See* pathogenic exercise.

Family Based Treatment (FBT), 106

Fat, 15, 25, 32, 36, 41, 56, 87, 88–89, 95

Fatigue, 4, 5, 24, 93, 116

and Compulsive Exercise, 68, 69, 70

and malnutrition, 96

in Anorexia Nervosa, 34, 42

in Bulimia Nervosa, 46, 49

in Female Athlete Triad, 70

Fiber, 90, 95

insoluble, 90

soluble, 90

Fully Recovered Stage, 108, 113–116

acceptance of self, 115

avoiding relapse, 113–114

body image, 114

exercise, 114

importance of daily choices, 115

requires periodic check-ups, 113

Functional magnetic resonance imaging (fMRI), 8

Gastroparesis, 6, 13, 14f, 15, 92
    connection to malnutrition, 15
    in Anorexia Nervosa, 34
    in Bulimia Nervosa, 52
Glucose, 6, 69, 89, 90
Gluten intolerance, 95-96
Harris-Benedict Formula, 24
Healthy eating, 86–87
    questions and answers for, 95–97
Higher Level of Care (HLOC), 98
    inpatient care, 102
    insurance coverage, 104
    intensive outpatient (IOP), 103
    necessity of, 101
    options if no insurance, 105
    options in, 102, 102f
    partial hospitalization (PHP), 103
    questions and answers for, 105–106
    residential treatment, 102–103
    selection of, 103–104
Hypermetabolic state, 21, 22, 24, 74
Hypertension, 56, 81
Hypoglycemia, 89
Hypometabolic state, 1, 2, 4, 5, 21, 22, 24, 25, 26, 27, 29, 32, 40, 48,
    49, 50, 56, 57, 58, 71, 72, 74, 78, 82, 84, 87, 91, 92, 94, 112
Illnesses that mimic / present as an eating disorder, 7
    gastrointestinal illnesses, 7
    endocrine disorders, 7
Indirect calorimetry, 22, 30
Insulin resistance, 96

Lack of energy. *See* fatigue.
Low blood glucose. *See* hypoglycemia.
Maudsley Approach. *See* Family Based Treatment.
Malnutrition, 1–4, 58, 86, 87, 96–97, 100, 116

and catabolic state, 4

and compulsive exercise, 63, 69

and eating disorders, 1, 3–4

and hypometabolic state, 4

and importance of serotonin, 8–9

and vulnerability to eating disorders, 11

at a young age, 39

body's adaptation to, 3, 4

cardiac complications in, 6

case study, 4–6

causes of, 3

cognitive problems, 8

compulsive thoughts, 8

gastrointestinal complaints, 6

identification of, 4–8

immune system damage, 7

in Anorexia Nervosa, 32, 33

in Binge Eating Disorder, 58

in Bulimia Nervosa, 46, 47

loss of protein matrix tissue, 6–7

low phase angle, 26

neurological and psychological changes and complications of, 2–3, 7–8

other physical complaints, 7

physiological effects of, 1, 2, 3, 4, 5, 6–7

treatment of, 20

usefulness of MT and BCA in, 9–10

Menstruation, 33, 42, 69, 70, 73, 119

Metabolic rate, 2, 20, 21, 29, 30, 40, 41, 42, 58, 71, 72, 74, 79, 82, 84, 90, 91, 92, 93, 94, 112, 119, 120

changing energy levels, with recovery, 94

correction of, with balanced eating, 92

measurement of, 22–23

Metabolic Testing (MT), 4, 9–10, 16, 19, 20, 22–26, 23f, 28, 30, 34, 36, 39, 40, 42, 50, 57, 58, 71, 72, 78, 79, 81, 82, 87, 90, 94, 100, 112, 120
    questions and answers for, 29–30
Metabolism, 5, 20–22, 24, 30, 40, 58, 71, 82, 91, 112, 114
    down-regulation, 24, 25
    effect of exercise on, 29
    improvement in, 29, 41, 93
    slow in, 1, 29, 40, 57, 58, 90, 92
Minnesota Starvation Experiment, 2–3
Mouth hunger, 51, 61, 93
Multivitamins, 96
Neurotransmitters, 9, 15, 65, 66
    levels of, 13, 14f, 54, 87, 111, 112, 113
Night Eating Syndrome, 76, 78
Nutrition, 86–87
    balanced food plan, 87–91
    what the body needs to function, 87
Nutritional assessment, complete, 19, 20, 86, 100
Obsessive-compulsive thoughts, 11, 12–13, 14f, 15, 18, 32, 110, 113
    during recovery, 112, 113
    evolution into eating disorder voice, 12–13
    in Anorexia Nervosa, 32, 39, 41, 42
    in Binge Eating Disorder, 55, 58,
    in OSFED, 80–81
    increase in with normal eating 16–17
Ongoing Recovery Stage, 108, 111–113
    and co-morbidities, 111
    and exercise, 112
    body image, 112–113
    intuitive eating, 112
Orthorexia Nervosa, 37
Osteopenia, 7
    and compulsive exercise, 69, 71
    in Anorexia Nervosa, 7, 39

Osteoporosis, 6, 73
    and compulsive exercise, 69, 70, 73
    in Anorexia Nervosa, 6
Other Specified Feeding and Eating Disorders (OSFED), 3, 75–76
    cardiac complications in, 81
    case study, 78–79
    disorders, 77–78
    gastrointestinal complaints, 81
    hiding of, 79–80
    neurological and psychological changes and complications of, 81–82
    other complications, 81
    physiological changes and complications of, 80
    questions and answers for, 84–85
    sub-types, 76–77
    treatment challenges, 79–80
    usefulness of MT and BCA in, 81–83
    weight loss help, 80
Outpatient treatment protocol, 99–100, 100f
    individualized treatment plan, 100–101
    initial treatment goals, 102
Pathogenic exercise, 64
Phase angle, 26, 30, 40, 119
Polycystic Ovary Syndrome (PCOS), 98
Predicted resting energy expenditure (PREE), 22, 25
Primary exercise dependence, 65
Protein, 7, 13, 15, 40, 41, 51, 57, 59, 60, 61, 78, 82, 84, 86, 87, 88, 89, 93, 95
    stores, 1, 4, 24, 25, 30, 82, 96, 114
    substrate utilization, 5, 25, 48
Psychotherapy, 18, 61, 102f, 109, 110, 111, 117
Psychotropic medication, 15–16
    connection to eating disorder voice, 15
Purging Disorder, 76, 78
    self-induced vomiting in, 78

Recovery, 107, 108, 119
  and alternative therapies, 117
  and denial, 118
  as process, 107–108
  better is not recovered, 108
  enhancing, 117–118
  outpatient treatment, 109–110
  questions and answers for, 117–118
  stages of, 108
Re-feeding edema, 9, 10, 29, 50, 52
Relative energy deficit in sports (REDS), 70,71
Resiliency, 116
Resting metabolic rate (RMR), 91
Secondary exercise dependence, 65
Semi-starvation, 2
Serotonin, 8–9, 13, 35, 42, 47, 62, 63, 65, 66, 109, 110, 111, 114, 116
Serotonin sensitivity, 9
Simple sugars. *See* carbohydrates, simple.
Sub-Threshold Bulimia Nervosa, 76, 77
Sub-Threshold Binge Eating Disorder, 76, 77–78
Sustained recovery, 109, 119–120
  components of, 119–120
  milestones in, 120–124
Starvation, 1, 2, 6, 10, 58, 82
  death from, 6
  in Anorexia Nervosa, 33
  in bariatric surgery patients, 37
  Minnesota Starvation Experiment, 2–3
  psychological effects of, 2–3
  physiological effects of, 2, 6, 10
Structured meal plan, 17
Testimonials, 121–124
Tiredness. *See* fatigue.
Total fat depletion, 6
Treatment protocol, 4, 24, 27, 28, 59, 86, 98, 99–100, 120

Treatment team, 98–99

Tryptophan, 13

Weight restoration, 8, 29, 30, 41, 101, 102, 102f, 103, 108, 113, 114

CPSIA information can be obtained
at www.ICGtesting.com
Printed in the USA
BVHW041102011218
534519BV00020B/734/P